Reviews of the previous edition:

'John Hamwee offers an eloquent description of this subtle and increasingly popular therapy.'

– Andrew Shields, Time Out

'Hamwee's writing style held my attention with such lightness, often at a deep level of lucid intellectual enquiry, that I read the book in a single sitting. Whether the reader is directly involved in Zero Balancing, or open to understanding its place in a wider movement, this book will likely prove illuminating and inspiring.'

– Caduceus

'This book is eminently readable...the writing is superbly elegant and concise and the brightness of [Hamwee's] humour carries one along with ease.'

– Richard Beaumont, Kindred Spirit, issue 50

zero
balancing

zero
balancing

TOUCHING THE ENERGY OF BONE

REPRINT EDITION

JOHN HAMWEE

Foreword by Fritz Smith, MD FCCAc
Illustrations by Gina Michaels

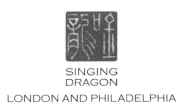

SINGING
DRAGON
LONDON AND PHILADELPHIA

This edition published in 2015
by Singing Dragon
an imprint of Jessica Kingsley Publishers
73 Collier Street
London N1 9BE, UK
and
400 Market Street, Suite 400
Philadelphia, PA 19106, USA

www.singingdragon.com

First published by Frances Lincoln, London, UK, 1999

Library of Congress Cataloging in Publication Data
Hamwee, John, author.
 Zero balancing : touching the energy of bone / John Hamwee ; foreword by Fritz Smith ;
illustrations by
Gina Michaels. -- Reprint edition.
    p. ; cm.
 Reprint of the original edition published in 1999 by Frances Lincoln.
 Includes bibliographical references and index.
 ISBN 978-1-84819-234-8
 I. Title.
 [DNLM: 1. Therapeutic Touch. 2. Bone and Bones--metabolism. 3. Energy Transfer. WB
890]
 RZ401
 615.8'52--dc23
                          2014013842

British Library Cataloguing in Publication Data
A CIP catalogue record for this book is available from the British Library

ISBN 978 1 84819 234 8
eISBN 978 0 85701 182 4

Printed and bound in Great Britain

for Dorsett

acknowledgements

Frances Lincoln received this book with enthusiasm and produced it beautifully. Jessica Kingsley has encouraged me as an author and acted in her usual prompt and decisive way with this edition. It has been my great good fortune to have had two such remarkable publishers.

Meriel Darby and Fritz Smith were my earliest teachers and I continue to explore the richness of what they gave me, many years ago now.

Cathy Bor, Deidre Burton, Kate Cave, Jake Chapman, Paul Cohen, Myra Connell, Scilla Elworthy, Hugh Miall and Felicity Wight all helped in different ways and improved the book immeasurably. Those who enjoy reading it can be very grateful to them, as I am.

contents

foreword

· ·

One of the major developments in health care in the past 40 years has been the introduction of Eastern ideas into Western thought. This Eastern influence has shown up in a number of ways: traditional Chinese medicine, acupuncture and Ayurvedic medicine as well as meditation, Yoga, T'ai Chi, Qi Gong and all the martial arts. A key aspect of this infusion centres on the introduction of energy as a specific force in nature and, for the purpose of Zero Balancing, a specific force within the human body.

Common themes run throughout these Eastern principles and practices. First is that the body and the mind form a single entity and cannot be treated separately. Second is an emphasis on harmony, balance and integration within this entity. These factors are not merely important to good health and a happy life – they are the very foundation of them. A third theme is the necessity of inner awareness and the fostering of those practices which address a person's internal environment. These include how to quiet the mind, clear and organize the body, and integrate the two into one well-functioning whole.

Zero Balancing is a hands-on therapy which works directly with this wisdom from the East, and integrates it with Western scientific and medical knowledge through the medium of conscious touch. Zero Balancing addresses specific symptoms and a client's complaints within a single session or a series of sessions. It also promotes greater harmony, balance and integration within the body and a better relationship – less scattered or chaotic – between the mind and body. Often it brings an experience of expanded awareness which enables greater peace, stillness and order. Clients often report significantly improved feelings of well-being on all levels – body, mind, emotion and spirit – and, in many cases, their lives seem to move forward more smoothly.

In *Zero Balancing: Touching the Energy of Bone*, John Hamwee, himself a practitioner and teacher of Zero Balancing, has presented an in-depth look into the therapy showing its development, theory, usage and outcomes. He explains how Eastern and Western views of health and healing are woven into its fabric. He expresses his passion for Zero Balancing and points the way for others to realize the potential of this work. This is an important and timely book. It defines a fascinating, growing edge of expanded health care possibilities. And it offers both health care practitioners and their clients new options in their quest for information and actualization.

Fritz Smith, MD FCCAc
Founder of Zero Balancing

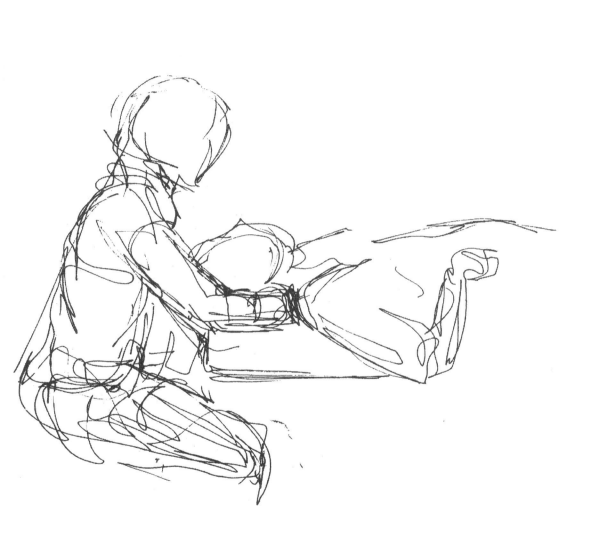

preface

· ·

The main aim of this book is to bring the principles and concepts of Zero Balancing to a wider audience than just those involved in health care. It is my passionate belief that these principles will enhance their work – whatever their professional practice – and that their patients and clients will benefit as a result. Regardless of whether or not these readers ever choose to become practitioners of Zero Balancing, its basic ideas are of immense importance to the whole business of serving those who come to them for help. Secondarily, I hope that the book will be useful to those learning or considering learning Zero Balancing, and to those clients who want to know what their practitioner is doing and why it works.

I want to emphasize that this book does not teach how to become a Zero Balancing practitioner. That is done at several workshops, separated by a period of practice, and is generally only open to those with a professional qualification in some form of health care. There is absolutely no substitute for this form of training led by a qualified instructor. Having said that, there is much that can be communicated, and much that can instruct, challenge, excite and inspire, through the written word.

This is a book about Zero Balancing – not the definitive book about it. I am aware that my fellow practitioners will not agree with everything that is in it, although I trust that they will think it is worthwhile. They will have their own view of Zero Balancing, and bring to it their own interests, background, perceptions and skills, as I have brought mine. There are many good books to be written about Zero Balancing, as there are about any interesting and mature therapy, and I very much hope that other books will be written. Thanks to the richness of Zero Balancing, there is certainly plenty of scope for them.

Throughout the book, for the sake of simplicity and consistency, I refer to the practitioner as 'she' and the client as 'he'.

This book could not have been written at all without the work of Fritz Frederick Smith MD, the originator of Zero Balancing. Practically all the ideas in it come from him; valuable and fascinating ideas which have, in my opinion, immensely wide applications. In addition I want to acknowledge that his great skills as a practitioner and teacher have inspired me, as they have inspired many others also, to learn and continue to learn about this remarkable form of bodywork. Those who find any part of this book interesting will be fascinated by his book *Inner Bridges*. It does not describe Zero Balancing, as this book does, but provides the background for everything that is here.

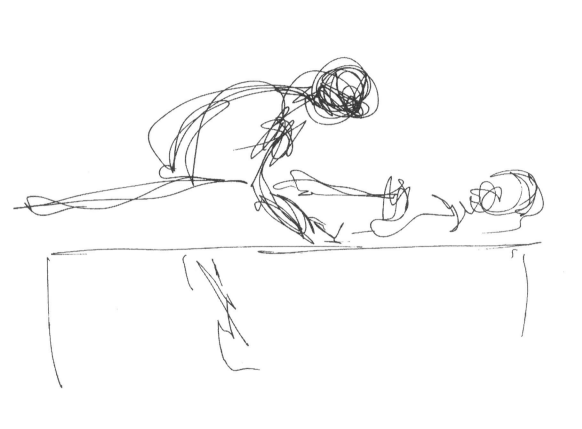

balance

· ·

Harriet has come for a Zero Balancing session. She doesn't look at all well, with pallid skin and deep rings under her eyes. She knows something isn't right but doesn't know what it is. A widow for 15 years, she has brought up her three children who have now left home and settled into their own lives. She is a grandmother, she loves her house and garden and is surrounded by good friends. She arranges flowers for a living. Life is good. And now, for no reason, she's not enjoying anything.

She is lying fully clothed on the couch in my treatment room. I sit at her head with my hands under her back, lifting gently. Suddenly a tear forms at the edge of her left eye; the next one pushes it away from her eyelash and it runs down her cheek. Then another. The room goes still and quiet. She is in some deep inner experience; we both hold our breath as if even to breathe might disturb the moment. Then she sighs. I ask her if all is well. 'I just feel sad, very sad', she replies. 'But it feels alright – in fact it feels good.'

Soon after, I bring the session to a close and as she gets up off the couch I can see that she has changed. Whatever it was that was disturbing her has gone. With a sense of discovery she recounts two long-forgotten incidents – being left at school and a boat trip in Paris the year after her husband died. Both are moments of grief and betrayal, and of feelings suppressed at the time. She is tired but at peace again, and her eyes have recovered their brightness.

Many of the key features of Zero Balancing are captured in this brief story. The work is done with the client lying fully clothed on a massage couch. It involves very gentle touch with no manipulation of bone or massaging of muscles. It can evoke deep emotion and long-forgotten memories. Clients look and feel much better after a session, whether their pain is physical, mental, spiritual or some combination of all of them. In fact, there is a sense in which something important has been resolved, even though they haven't analysed or discussed what was the matter in the first place.

The first time I watched a Zero Balancing session, in which something similar happened to the client, it seemed like magic. I couldn't imagine what the practitioner was doing that could be having such a powerful effect, so I assumed that it was some innate skill of his which could not be explained or taught to anyone else. As I was to discover, that is not the case. The work is based on a clear and communicable theory about the human body, and the procedures which the practitioner uses can be learned relatively quickly. Even novices can get remarkable results; and those with many years' experience get them more reliably and with a wider range of problems and issues.

The more I learned about Zero Balancing the more I came to see some of its wider implications. Its core theories, concepts, and techniques open up many possibilities for helping people; possibilities which can be turned into simple, practical work. And, as I relate in Chapter 7, I also think that these core ideas form part of a wider movement, amounting to a re-perception of illness and healing, which will have a profound effect on the practice of medicine in the future.

Zero Balancing started over 20 years ago. Fritz Smith, its originator, trained as an osteopath and later qualified as a doctor. He had a varied general practice in a small rural town and also worked in the local hospital. There were perhaps two things that marked him out as different from his medical colleagues. One was that he placed great emphasis on touching his patients in a way that felt safe and comfortable to them. To some extent this may have come from his training as an osteopath, although he attributes more importance to the fact that his father was a renowned chiropractor and that, as a child, he enjoyed his father's skilled touch.

The other difference between Fritz Smith and his colleagues was his open mindedness. For example, in the early 1970s he attended a short course given by an acupuncturist. One treatment in particular made a powerful impression. The patient was an elderly man who could not open his right hand; it had been involuntarily clenched for some time. The acupuncturist had inserted a needle into a point just below his left knee, and the hand opened. I imagine that most doctors witnessing a treatment of this kind, especially at a time when acupuncture was far less respected in the West than it is now, would have dismissed it in some way. Fritz himself says that he has always been grateful that the acupuncture point chosen was not in or near the hand itself; if it had been, he might have been satisfied with a Western medical explanation for what had happened – perhaps the needle had hit, and reactivated, a trapped nerve. Instead he appreciated that the anatomy and physiology he had been taught at medical school were incomplete descriptions of how the human body works.

Another example comes from Fritz Smith's book *Inner Bridge*s. He examined a man both before, and immediately after, a firewalk over 20 feet of burning hot coals. After the walk, 'His feet had ashes on them, but they were cool to the touch, slightly sweaty, and free from any signs of burns or blisters...' (Fritz Frederick Smith MD, *Inner Bridges*, p. 21). Again, instead of regarding this as some one-off freakish phenomenon, Fritz Smith took it seriously. Whatever the explanation, he accepted that it could not be found within the framework of Western medicine.

To learn more about phenomena such as these, he qualified and practised as an acupuncturist, combining it with osteopathic manipulation. His practice was a busy one and he knew that what he was doing worked well for his patients, but his inquiring mind wanted to understand more. How could the different traditions of Eastern and Western medicine be reconciled? What he had learned about energy, from acupuncture, must be consistent in some way with what he had learned about anatomy, from osteopathy, and what he had learned about physiology from his medical training. It wasn't that one was right and the others wrong; they were all true, and all partially true. Was there some theory which could unite them, some form of treatment which could make use of them all?

A few years later, he did indeed find what he was looking for, and this book describes and explains what he discovered. For some time his clinical work, based on that discovery, didn't have a name – it was just what he did. Then, one day, a patient came up off the couch after one of his treatments and said, 'I feel balanced...back to Zero' (meaning back to how she was before all the stresses and strains of life had taken their toll) '...sort of Zero Balanced.' The name stuck. At the time of writing, some 40 years later, there are over 1500 qualified practitioners of Zero Balancing, about 100 of whom are also qualified to teach it at over 50 workshops each year, and there are countless clients who have benefited from it.

All these practitioners work in the way that Fritz Smith developed and is still developing. Following a basic procedure, which takes about half an hour to complete and which is described later in this book, they use gentle traction, or gentle finger pressure at various places on the trunk, legs, neck and feet. The pressure is not on acupuncture points, nor is its effect on the muscles of the body – distinguishing Zero Balancing from Shiatsu, and other forms of acupressure on the one hand, and from massage, Rolfing and forms of bio-energetics on the other. The traction and pressure are both directed to the bones and joints underlying soft tissue – but, in contrast to osteopathy and chiropractic, there is no manipulation of those bones and joints. As with cranio-sacral therapy, it works with both the structure and the energy of the body, but its concern is not with one particular mechanism, rather with the organization of the body as a whole. Anyone who has experienced any of these kinds of bodywork, and then has a Zero Balancing session, notices the differences immediately.

Introducing Zero Balancing in this way, as the invention of one man, and with its own distinctive characteristics, emphasizes its uniqueness. In the next few chapters, in order to explain what Zero Balancing is and how it works, I write about it as if it were unique. However, it is also the case that Fritz Smith was working at a time and in a culture in which complementary therapies were gaining increasing recognition, and a number of new therapies were being developed. Many of them have much in common, and it is interesting to look at what they share. If large numbers of complementary practitioners are all doing effective work which, however different the techniques they use, has a common basis, then investigation of that common basis may well tell us something important about illness, health and healing. Chapter 7 looks at Zero Balancing in this context. For now, I want to start with a concept much used by complementary therapies – the concept of balance.

In general, good health is seen as the maintenance of a state of balance, and illness or dysfunction is seen as the consequence of some imbalance. Zero Balancing uses this idea too, but in a precise and specific way. It is based on the view that, in health, there is a well-functioning balance between body structure and body energy. In a moment I will explain fully what is meant by body structure and body energy. For now I want to point out that there are plenty of everyday examples of the basic distinction between structure and energy. The structure of a tree is its roots, trunk and branches. And all of that structure needs energy from the sun to grow. Similarly, the engine and body of a car can be seen as its structure, but without the energy provided by fuel it's just an inert heap of metal. More abstractly, organizations have structures – that is established patterns of communication, control and responsibility – but without the energy of employees working through those structures, nothing much happens.

We can perceive the human body in the same way. Roughly speaking, its structure is its physical form and energy is what animates it. The core of Zero Balancing concerns the relationship between structure and energy in the body; a very specific relationship which will become clear after I have discussed structure and energy separately.

. . . .

structure

Structure is a relative term; it means that which is relatively stable and enduring. So in common speech it can mean a whole building or, to an architect or engineer it can mean that part of the building which forms its core or frame; distinguishing it, for example, from windows and internal walls. Given that it is a relative term, what is considered as stable and enduring depends on some implicit comparison. A stable relationship between two businesses may be one which has lasted only a few years, but a good deal longer than most; a stable marriage may have lasted decades.

The most stable and enduring part of the body is bone. It is by far the most dense tissue, it changes its shape (within limits) more slowly than any other tissue, and it lasts long after death. So when I talk about structure in Zero Balancing, I'm talking about bone, and about the skeleton – a set of bones connected by joints. Zero Balancing sees the skeleton as one unit, one thing – with many parts, certainly – but still, as a whole.

Why? Why does it not simply work on a foot, for example, or the neck if that is the area which is not working well? The root answer is that Zero Balancing is a system of healing; but that answer won't make much sense until I've explained a little more.

Look first at the skeleton purely as at a piece of engineering. Imagine you have twisted your right ankle and walk, for a week or two, in such a way as to protect it and prevent pain. You might notice, for example, that in order to do so, you splay your foot out more than usual as you move. That works fine, but after a while you may find that your knee is complaining a bit – knees work best when they hinge straight, and if your splayed-out foot introduces a slight twist in the knee, the misalignment of bones and the unequal stress on the ligaments on each side will start to become apparent as discomfort or even pain. So you find a way of walking which protects the knee, and that introduces a distortion in the hip joint above. And so on and so on. And all this without even considering the effect of putting more weight than usual on your left leg – in order to protect the right. It is clear that any local problem will have widespread effects.

In this example, I describe a pattern of walking which lasted a few weeks; at least as common are patterns of using the body which last many, many years. One client, in her mid-fifties, with whom I worked over an extended period, had chronic intermittent pain in her feet and back. After a number of sessions she realized that the root cause was that as a child she was expected to be self-effacing. She grew up in a very large house where children were supposed to be seen and not heard. She responded to this, instinctively, by tip-toeing as she walked, and carried on doing so all through her adult life even though the original reason for this behaviour had long since passed. To heal the chronic and intermittent pain, all the resulting distortions to her skeleton had to be addressed.

All this is to say that while there is a simple, mechanical reason for treating the skeleton as a whole, there is also a more complex emotional reason. There are a number of common phrases that link bone with deep emotional issues: 'I feel it in my bones,' 'What's bred in the bone' or 'Bone-tired.' Maybe there is a wisdom in these phrases; perhaps it is in bone that we store deep knowledge, and deep responses to our experiences. It is worth adding here that it is an assumption of modern Western culture that we only know things in our mind, which is in our brain, which is in our head. This is an assumption, not a fact. There is no proof that this is how or where we store all knowledge. Other cultures see it differently. Chinese, for example, has a term – *Hsin Hsin* – which is normally translated as 'the heart-mind'. It is that part of our knowing and thinking which resides in, and comes from, the heart. (Actually, *Hsin Hsin* can't really be translated at all precisely because, in this culture, we don't regard the heart as capable of thought.)

Western biochemistry research is also challenging the traditional assumption that it is only in the brain that we know things. Candace Pert, Research Professor in the Department of Physiology and Biophysics at Georgetown University Medical Centre, Washington, writes, 'Originally, we scientists thought that the flow of neuropeptides and receptors was being directed from centres in the brain...as a result of my own and other people's work in the laboratory, we found...we then had to consider a system with intelligence diffused throughout, rather than a one way operation adhering strictly to the laws of cause and effect, as was previously thought when we believed that the brain ruled over all' (Candace Pert, *Molecules of Emotion*, p. 310).

There is a good deal of evidence that memories of certain kinds of trauma are stored in the bone. Quite often in a Zero Balancing session, touch at a particular place on a bone will evoke long-forgotten memories. Most obviously, clients will remember an injury or fracture, and may make an association between that trauma and a current problem. Less frequent, but still relatively common, is the recollection of an emotional trauma, as in the story at the start of this chapter. One client I worked with is a Jungian therapist, a woman who had spent many years in therapy herself. During a Zero Balancing session, to help with the migraines from which she had suffered for many years, she suddenly remembered an incident in her childhood. It was of her mother's glance at a man who was in her house. A glance of fear mixed with desire. It shocked the child, and made her feel a complex mixture of emotions: distrust of her mother, insecurity at the threat to the family, loyalty towards her father, anger that he wasn't there, and so on. The point is that this incident, these emotions, had not surfaced before, but came into consciousness through touch on bone.

One final example comes from my own first Zero Balancing session as a client of Fritz Smith. As he worked on my right foot, I became aware of myself as a very small baby, and of the experience of starving, of trying to feed but not receiving nourishment. I didn't know if it was what had happened to me, or if it was some kind of hallucination – but with his help, by way of an experiment, I took it for real and managed to feel compassion for myself and my mother, and to let go of feelings of anger and frustration. I checked with my mother later and she told me that it was indeed true. She had been exhausted at the end of the war, when I was born, and although she thought she was feeding me I continued to lose weight. After many weeks, it was discovered that she had no milk. I have absolutely no idea why this memory was held in my right foot – but I have no doubt that it was.

Fritz Smith's explanation for this bone-held memory is a hypothesis. He suggests that normally we are able react to trauma – we recoil from a blow, the soft tissue of the muscles absorbs some of the shock and bounces back. When cruel, angry or unkind words are hurled at us, we answer back or we argue, either openly or silently, that the comment is unfair or inaccurate. All these responses serve to prevent the trauma hurting us deep within and lodging there. However, there are times when we cannot react. We may be too frightened to respond or unaware of the mental pain we have experienced; we may be unconscious or simply so young that we don't know what is happening. In these instances, he argues, the shock goes to the bone. And, in ways I explain later, it leaves its mark there.

So far I have looked at mechanical and emotional reasons for working on the whole skeleton. There is a further reason too; a reason which takes us into the domain of energy.

· ·

energy

There is a good deal of unnecessary mystification surrounding this concept; and a good deal of unproductive suspicion. In fact, we all know energy perfectly well.

We know what it feels like when we can't wait to do some task we've been looking forward to, or go sailing on a sunny day, or climb a hill which has a good view. And we all know what it feels like when we are weary and depressed, can hardly drag ourselves into or out of bed; or when we droop because we haven't eaten for a long time. And we know how quickly we can flip from one to the other; the times when we've been lifted out of lethargy by unexpected good news or the arrival of a loved one.

Western medical research seeks explanations for these kinds of phenomena in levels, and changes in levels, of body chemistry; and there is no doubt that there are correlations between some of these experiences and body chemistry changes. I don't need to get into a discussion about what causes what – whether body chemistry changes energy levels, or vice versa, or indeed, if there is some deeper cause which changes both energy levels and body chemistry together. Whatever the cause, there is no doubting the everyday experience which we call energy.

The Eastern world has investigated the phenomena of energy for many thousands of years – not so much from the standpoint of trying to find causes, but with a view to understanding its anatomy – how and where it flows in the body. What has emerged are coherent accounts which describe an energy body much as Western anatomy and physiology describe the physical body. These descriptions of the energy body are good ones; good, because therapies based on them have proved effective. The best known example is acupuncture anaesthesia.

> Films were shown of surgeries being performed. A cancerous lung was removed, the only anaesthesia being an acupuncture needle in each of the patient's ears and another in each arm,

27

manually stimulated by the attending acupuncturist. The film showed a patient having a brain tumour excised with the aid of an acupuncture needle inserted in the forearm... Throughout each procedure the patients were awake, talking, and even occasionally taking sips of water. At the conclusion of one surgery the patient sat up on the table and shook hands with his doctor and the attending staff. In another case, after the removal of a thyroid tumour, the patient actually stepped down from the operating table and walked to the wheelchair by himself. (Fritz Frederick Smith MD, *Inner Bridges*, p. 17)

Having said all that, the question remains – what is this energy in the body? It is clear from this example that it isn't just a matter of faith. No one could suppose that acupuncture anaesthesia works because patients believe in it. In any case it works on animals too – who, presumably, don't believe in it. However, research into what it is has not been successful. Over some of the traditional locations of acupuncture points there are indeed detectable electrical differences on the skin compared to other locations, suggesting that this energy is some kind of electrical current. But that doesn't hold true for many acupuncture points. Similarly, suggestions that acupuncture treatment stimulates endorphin releases haven't been satisfactorily validated either. In fact, I don't know of any satisfactory answer to this question of what it is.

That may be because it isn't a good question. It really goes back to Fritz Smith's realization that there was something here that could not be explained in terms of Western medical physiology, or indeed Western language and concepts. The concept of Qi – of which the word 'energy' is a rough translation – is a part of the Chinese culture, underlying a host of attitudes and practices from Feng Shui to medicine, from diet to T'ai Chi. If I were Chinese, I could probably answer the question; but you'd have to be Chinese too to understand the answer!

However, like countless others, I can feel something – something which I can use the word 'energy' to describe. When I receive a Zero Balancing session, for example, I may feel as if part of my body has been activated, and I didn't realize it was inactive until that happened. Sometimes I feel a wave passing from one part of my body to another; occasionally the wave flows right through me. Sometimes I feel a sudden warmth in a particular area. And in all these cases, I may feel the change quite a long way away from where the practitioner is working. Also, when I am working as a practitioner I can feel a sensation of movement and flow under my fingers, and if I touch the client's hand the skin will often feel warmer, smoother and softer than before. Usually the effect isn't local. That is, after having felt a change in one place I find a change elsewhere in the body too. As far as I am concerned, what I am feeling is the same as is reported by many others – acupuncturists, Qi Gong practitioners, cranio-sacral therapists, meditators and others – and which we all call energy.

I cover this further in Chapter 2. For now, all that is necessary is that you have some idea of what I am talking about when I use the word energy. And that you are prepared to accept, for now, that it is a phenomenon which, although unexplained, is real.

I have referred a lot to acupuncture because it is a well-established system of medicine. As such, it provides evidence that there is an anatomy of energy: patterns of organized energy flow in the body. However, this energy anatomy is concerned largely with the flow of energy in the soft tissue of the body and is not directly relevant to Zero Balancing, which is concerned with bone and the skeleton. Fritz Smith's understanding, which is shared by a number of other complementary therapies, is that energy also flows through bone. He suggests that this is because human beings are essentially vertical structures.

You can have a subjective experience of the flow of energy through a vertical structure. Stand directly under the spire of a church or cathedral, and it is a remarkable sensation. It is not easy to describe, but the best I can do is to say that it is a feeling of focus; as if all the separate parts of you are lined up harmoniously. I am reminded too of experiments with magnets which I was shown at school. I was given a tray of iron filings, with different sizes and shapes scattered at random, muddled and messy, and with no pattern to them. Then I approached the tray, slowly, with a magnet. At the moment when the force field of the magnet was strong enough they fell instantaneously into a wonderful, magical pattern. With two magnets, each approaching the tray from a different direction, the instant pattern was more complex – that of two fields interacting. The magic, of course, was that I couldn't discern the magnet's force field with my own senses; but once it was registered by the filings, there it was in all its regularity and beauty. A glimpse into a hidden world. Now, when I feel the flow of energy through the church spire, down through my own body to the earth, it seems as though all the 'filings' that make up my own body have become aligned to some hidden pattern.

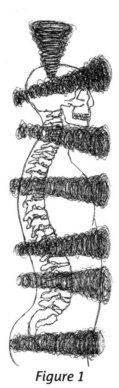

Figure 1

This vertical flow permeates the whole body, but it is at its most powerful and organized as it flows through the densest tissue: bone. The evidence for this comes from combining two observations. One is the repeated experience of those who have trained themselves to turn their attention most acutely to the inner rhythms and flows of the body, that there are seven vortices of energy – called chakras – in the body. The location of the chakras, and the quality of energy in each of them, is commonly agreed (Figure 1). As the figure indicates, the chakras are thought of as swirling, operating, in the soft tissue of the body.

The other observation was Fritz Smith's: 'One day in a Zero Balancing class as I was lecturing on skeletal anatomy and pointing out the normal curves of the spine, it suddenly occurred to me that, as the current of energy flows through the spine and around the spinal bends, as I believe it does, vortices of energy would be created at the major curves. As I studied the skeleton and imagined these vortices whirling, I recalled the picture of a meditating yogi with the overlay of the spinal chakras, and instinctively I knew the chakras must exist. They were not just abstract symbols of an ancient religious system; they actually corresponded to the structure of the human skeletal system...' (Fritz Frederick Smith MD, *Inner Bridges*, p. 49).

As far as I am aware, until Fritz Smith turned his attention to this issue, no one thought to relate the location of the chakras to the shape of the skeleton. In a moment of great insight, a moment which bridged Eastern and Western views of the world, he suddenly saw that relationship.

If you think of a river, and the way the flow creates circular eddies at the bends, this insight makes perfect sense. A flow is a flow. A flow of energy will have the same underlying pattern as a flow of water. There is support for this idea from Chinese medicine too. The energy channels which flow through soft tissue are almost always referred to as rivers, and the names of a host of acupuncture points refer to this idea too – for example, 'Returning current' and 'Greater mountain stream'. In the present context, what is most significant about this insight into the location of the chakras is that it provides support for the notion that energy flows through bone – in this instance, through the whole length of the spine.

So the most basic proposition of energy anatomy which is relevant to Zero Balancing is that energy flows through the bone and joints of the skeleton. As a consequence, it makes sense to work not just on a selected area, perhaps where the client feels pain or restriction of movement, but on the whole flow throughout the whole skeleton.

balancing

The basic theory of Zero Balancing can now be stated quite simply. The skeleton is one functional unit through which energy flows in an organized way. As we will see, from that simple sentence there unfolds a wonderful array of concepts, techniques, possibilities and insights.

Imagine a skeleton in which all the bones are in the correct relationship with each other. The femur, for example, sits in the hip socket with an even layer of cushioning between it and the bone of the pelvis. The ligaments which hold it in place and limit its range of motion are all evenly tensioned and there are no abnormalities of bone to restrict its easy movement as it rotates internally and externally. Structurally, it works perfectly, and it is easy to imagine that energy will flow freely and easily through the joint and on down the leg.

Take the rather more complex example, of a costo-vertebral joint, where a rib is attached to the spine (Figure 2). The three attachments of the rib to the spine make for stability – much as a camera tripod provides a stable base for the camera. They also provide flexibility. There is play in each of the three joints, so a considerable variety of movement is possible. In fact, this flexibility is essential. With each breath, the rib moves in three ways. It lifts, it extends outwards, and it rotates along its axis; all three of these movements are essential to full and healthy breathing. Again, if the joint is working perfectly, it is easy to imagine the flow of energy down the spine branching off and flowing through the joint and smoothly down the rib.

Now imagine that the joint, for whatever reason, has lost its flexibility at one, two or all three places where it attaches to the spine. Now, on an in-breath, the rib will be held tight and will not move in the ways I have mentioned. If this were your rib, you probably wouldn't even notice this restriction, and you would just live with it. What would happen over time? The answer is that the rib would develop extra layers of bone at a particular place. The best way of understanding this is to simulate the problem yourself.

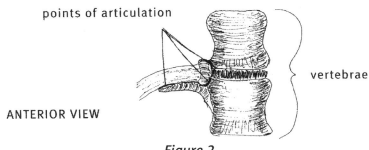

points of articulation

vertebrae

ANTERIOR VIEW

Figure 2

Find a curved green stick – that is, one with some resilience in it. With one hand, hold one end loosely between three fingers – a rough representation of the costo-vertebral joint. With your other hand, on the other end of the stick, make the movements of lifting, opening and rotating, and you will find that they are easy to do. Now grip one end of the stick tightly in your fist, simulating restriction in the costo-vertebral joint, and repeat the three movements. You can feel tremendous tension in the stick – and, in particular, you will feel that the tension is most powerfully focused in the area where the stick starts to curve. In the language of Zero Balancing, this is an area of held energy. In engineer's language, there is extra stress on the bone at that point, and the body responds, sensibly enough, by growing extra layers of bone just there to reinforce the point of greatest stress.

So there is a direct relationship between energy and structure. A change in the structure – in this case a restriction in the costo-vertebral joint – leads to changes in energy flows along the rib, which in turn lead to changes in the structure of the rib. In this example, I have described an initial change in structure which sets off the inter-related changes in energy and structure. But it could have been a disturbance in the energy flow along the spine that caused the structural problem in the costo-vertebral joint. Sometimes it is obvious which came first – the structural change or the energetic – and I will give examples of each in a moment. More often, I suspect it is really akin to the scenario of the chicken and the egg.

You can, if you want, ignore either one of these aspects. You can choose to work only with structure – as do most osteopaths and orthopaedic surgeons – and you can have good results on that basis. Or you can choose to work only with energy – as do most acupuncturists and Reiki practitioners – and that can be very effective too. But there is the intriguing possibility of bearing both aspects in mind simultaneously, and doing work on that basis. What would that look like? What kind of effects might that have?

I want to start my answer to these questions with the experience of a client who had broken her arm in a car crash 18 months before I saw her. The fracture had healed perfectly – according to the X-rays – but she still felt pain at the site of the injury, and was unable to use her arm to drive or do other normal activities. After a single Zero Balancing session she regained normal use of her arm. Looking at her injury as simply structural couldn't explain either why she was still having trouble after the fracture had healed or how such a gentle form of bodywork, involving no manipulation, could have had such a dramatic effect. Before going into more details of this example, I want to refer to the findings of a recent piece of research.

> X-rays and MRI scans of the spines of two groups of patients were taken; one group without pain and with normal freedom of movement, the other group composed of people immobilized by acute back pain. The pictures were then arranged randomly, and doctors were asked to identify which patients would be suffering from back pain. There was absolutely no correlation between the patients' experience and the doctors' diagnoses. That is, large numbers of people whose spines looked as if they would be the cause of agonising pain or severe lack of mobility reported no problem at all; and large numbers whose spines – structurally speaking – looked normal were in acute pain. (Andrew Weil MD, *Spontaneous Healing*, p. 120)

It is in cases like these that the idea of balancing energy and structure provides both a plausible explanation for what has happened and a way of resolving the problems caused. Take first the example of a person whose spine is distorted, structurally, but who feels no pain or restriction.

It may be that the energy flow has adapted to the structure as shown in Figure 3. It is easy to imagine that with a clear and consistent flow of energy not only will the spine itself function adequately, in spite of the distortions, but that energy will flow freely through the costo-vertebral joints and the ribs, enabling them to function adequately too. And if they are working reasonably well, the muscles which attach to the ribs won't be put under too much stress either; in other words, there are only small knock-on effects from the misalignment of the vertebrae of the spine. To use the language of Zero Balancing, energy and structure are balanced.

Now take the case of a person whose structure seems fine but who is complaining of symptoms. Figure 4 shows what may have happened to the client whose arm was broken. I have given three examples of the kinds of disturbances which can occur in the flow of energy along the bone. Generally speaking, an experienced practitioner can tell the difference between these by the feeling of the bone under her fingers. In all three examples, the point is that there is a lack of consistency between the healed state of the structure and the unhealed state of the energy flow – they are not in balance.

The same principle applies in the rather more complex case of the spine. Figure 5 gives some examples of what may have happened to the energy flow in the cases of those patients whose structure seemed fine but who were in pain. What could have caused these kinds of disturbances? With (a) and (b) it is possible that there was some kind of blow to the fourth vertebra from the top, or to the rib which is attached to it, which has disturbed the energy flow but not the structure. I am thinking of the kind of shock I had when I went down a step without realizing it was there. I felt a jarring, and most unpleasant it was too, in my spine. But when I had it checked later no vertebra had been displaced. Still, given the impact I felt, I wouldn't be surprised if there was some disruption of the energy flow through the spine. I suspect too that in the case of emotional shocks, although there is not necessarily any distortion of structure, there is a direct effect on energy. Receiving bad news can feel like a body blow. Being betrayed can feel like a stab in the back. I don't think it is fanciful to suppose that these feelings result from an impact not on the structural body but on the energy body, and leave their mark there. I have in mind too Fritz Smith's view that if a person is unable to respond immediately to the shock, its impact is received in the bone. As the bone is not distorted structurally by such emotional shocks, I take this to mean that the shock disturbs the energy flows in the bone.

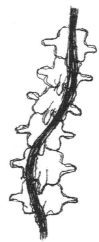

Figure 3

SITE OF FRACTURE AND DIRECTION OF IMPACT

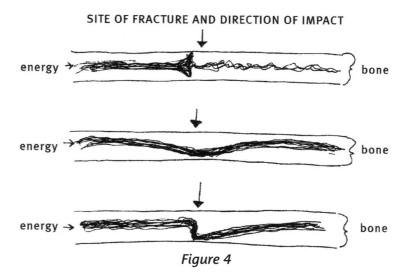

Figure 4

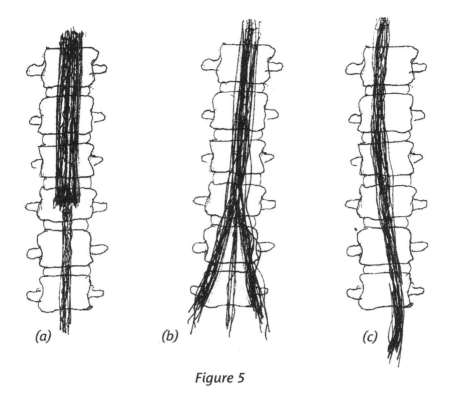

(a)   *(b)*   *(c)*

Figure 5

All this applies, though perhaps less obviously, to example (c) in Figure 5. Because of the gradual curve of the energy flow it seems unlikely that there has been a sudden localized shock, either physical or emotional. More probably, some relatively small but chronic disturbance has built up over a long time, each tiny change reinforcing the one that has gone before. The basic point, however, remains the same. A person whose energy and structure are out of balance with one another is likely to feel some effects – it may be as strong as acute pain or as mild as a long-term, gradually increasing, lack of mobility. And, although working with structure may re-establish the flows of energy, or working with energy may re-establish the alignment of structure, it makes sense, in these cases, to work with the two together.

This basic point holds true even when there are no obvious or disturbing symptoms. For many people, much of the time, the body finds some way of accommodating change. Watch almost any adult over the age of 40 just walking normally and you will see how one shoulder is held a little higher than the other, one foot splays out more than the other, perhaps the left side is a little turned in compared to the right. All this without any pain or problem. But the absence of pain or problems is a very limited goal, and not the same as the enjoyment of full health; rather as the absence of war is not the same as peace. Like Harriet, whose story started this chapter, we are so often unaware that we are coping rather than living. Rebalancing a person's energy and structure, bringing them 'back to Zero', can bring about profound changes for the better, even if that person felt all right or was managing before. It can lead to a tremendous increase in potential: the potential to undertake things previously thought too difficult, to choose fulfilling work or relationships, to enjoy life to the full. That is the true promise of balancing structure and energy.

touch

· ·

At last he takes her hand, raising it in both of his own. Now he bends over the bed in a kind of crouching stance, his head drawn down into the collar of his robe. His eyes are closed as he feels for her pulse. In a moment he has found the spot, and for the next half-hour he remains thus, suspended over the patient like some exotic golden bird with folded wings, holding the pulse of the woman beneath his fingers, cradling her hand in his. All the power of the man seems to have been drawn down into this one purpose. It is palpation of the pulse raised to the state of ritual. From the foot of the bed, where I stand, it is as though he and the patient have entered a special place of isolation, of apartness, about which a vacancy hovers, and across which no violation is possible. After a moment the woman rests back upon her pillow. From time to time she raises her head to look at the strange figure above her, then sinks back once more. I cannot see their hands joined in a correspondence that is exclusive, intimate, his fingertips receiving the voice of her sick body through the rhythm and throb she offers at her wrist. All at once I am envious – not of him, not of Yeshi Dhonden for his gift of beauty and holiness, but of her. I want to be held like that, touched so, received...

As he nears the door, the woman raises her head and calls to him in a voice at once urgent and serene. 'Thank you, doctor,' she says, and touches with her other hand the place he had held on her wrist, as though to recapture something that had visited there. (Ram Dass and Paul Gorman, *How Can I Help?*, p. 119)

This chapter is concerned with how structure and energy can be balanced. The simple answer is through touch. However, not just any old touch will do – it has to have specific qualities.

This may seem a little strange. Either you are touching someone or you aren't. Where does quality come in? It is, in fact, a common experience that one person's touch feels better than another's, but it is rare that anyone explores this interesting phenomenon. It is simply assumed to be a given, or something to do with the relationship between the two people concerned. But the quality of a person's touch is not immutable or invariant – anyone can learn to use different kinds of touch for different situations, and anyone can learn to use the kind of touch used in Zero Balancing. This kind of touch is essential for balancing structure and energy.

. . . .

interface

Interface touch is a very simple idea – one of those ideas about which, the first time you hear it, you tend to say, 'Oh yes, I see', and carry on as before. But if you really understand it, then a lifetime of learning and possibilities open up before you. The idea is that it is possible to touch another person while maintaining a clear boundary, or interface, between the two of you. At all times during the touch, you know where your body ends and the other person's begins – and the other person knows the same too.

I want to distinguish interface touch from other kinds of touch we commonly encounter. The kind of touch we are used to in intimate relationships is one which blurs the boundaries between two people. As babies, cradled in our mother's arms, most of us had the blissful experience of melting into her, of being 'one flesh'. Similarly, the pleasure of losing awareness of one's physical form and merging with a loved one is an important part of the joy of a sexual union. In these situations we lose our separateness, for a few moments, and the pain of loneliness is assuaged. A simple word for this kind of touch is 'blending'.

The physical bodies of the two people concerned do not literally blend, in the way that eggs and oil blend in a mayonnaise. But it is true to say that their energies do. That is, when this kind of touch is used, there has been some mingling of the two energy bodies; and the longer it is used, the deeper the effect. This explains why it can be so distressing to have this kind of touch from someone you don't like, or when it is inappropriate to the relationship between you. You don't want to have your energy body affected, altered, by the inclusion in it of some aspect of that other person – but it is happening all the same. It also explains, at least in part, the very painful sensation of loss when there is a separation from a loved one by death or divorce. Your energy body has become used to blending with theirs, and it feels vulnerable, wounded, incomplete, without that contact with the other.

This kind of touch can be used therapeutically. It can comfort a person in pain or distress, and it can provide a practitioner with information which she couldn't easily get in any other way. There are many reports that with this kind of touch it is possible to feel another person's pain – quite directly – and diagnose illnesses and complaints which have evaded discovery by more conventional methods. Therapeutically, this kind of touch can also be abused – a patient touched in this way may respond, instinctively and unconsciously, with feelings of intimacy, love, or sexual attraction for the practitioner. Such feelings arise from the touch itself – and perhaps what is evoked by the touch – and the client may well not realize what is happening, nor would he necessarily give his consent to it if he did know.

There is another kind of touch we are also familiar with. It can happen even with a simple handshake or a hug, although the effects are more noticeable with longer contact. It is a touch which leaves us feeling either revitalized or depleted. The reason it can have one of two opposite effects is that it is a touch which transmits energy from one person to the other. Sometimes you receive energy, so you feel revitalized: sometimes your energy is pulled into the other person and you feel low afterwards. In both cases what is happening is that one person's energy is 'streaming' into the other. Again, this touch is used therapeutically. A sign that it is being used is when the client feels better after a session and the practitioner feels drained.

Although some skilled practitioners can work with this kind of touch very deliberately, and indeed protect themselves from exhaustion, these kind of transfers most often take place unconsciously.

Neither of these kinds of touch – blending or streaming – maintains a clear and inviolate boundary between the two people involved. With both of them there is an interchange across the boundary of the physical and energy bodies. There is nothing intrinsically good or bad about such an interchange – as I have pointed out, it can be very beneficial or very damaging – everything depends on the circumstances. But neither touch can be used for Zero Balancing. There is a simple reason for this. The therapy works by balancing the client's own body structure with the client's own body energy. So any involvement of the practitioner's energy will just get in the way of that process. In addition, if there are energy transfers going on, the practitioner will get muddled about what is happening to whom. So she will find it hard to assess when the client's energy and structure aren't in balance, won't be sure about what has to be done to bring them into balance, and won't know when to stop working because they have become balanced. She won't get the kind of clear information which you get from an interface touch. The clarity comes from maintaining that boundary between the practitioner and client at all times. The next three sections talk about the qualities of an interface touch.

attention

When you drive your car, you can listen to the radio, plan what you are going to say at a meeting, talk to a companion, or daydream, while at the same time working out how soon and how much you need to brake to get round a corner, measuring the amount you have to turn the wheel (which is related to the speed you are going) and so on. A series of complex computations are carried out without you even being aware that you are doing them. The point here is that most of the time we touch we do so in the same way as we drive a car: the main focus of our attention is elsewhere.

Right now – as a small experiment – take your attention to your fingertips, wherever they are resting. As you do so, I expect you will suddenly become aware of the surface which they are touching. I bet that you were unaware of the feel, the texture, the heat or coldness of that surface before your attention was directed to your fingertips, and that you are now. Try running your fingers along that surface, and notice any changes in it. As I write, I'm doing this on a desk and I can feel the grain of the wood, and a spot which feels a bit strange. I look down, and it is a knot in the wood. It looks like a vortex, like an eddy in a river. Perhaps what I am feeling is a bit like the area of stress on a rib, which I mentioned in Chapter 1, a place where a disturbance in the energy flow has changed the structure.

Now – this bit is more difficult – try leaving your hand where it is and deliberately taking your attention away from it. Think of something you have to do, some problem you're facing. Of course, the difficulty is the same as when someone says to you 'Don't think about an elephant' – and you somehow can't stop yourself thinking about an elephant. It just forces its way into your mind. But, with a bit of luck, thinking about an elephant may have distracted your attention for a moment or two from the sensation under your fingertips. So, looking back at that moment when your attention was distracted from your fingertips, what do you notice about it?

The obvious thing is that you weren't picking up information any more. And that's a good enough reason in itself why a key quality of interface touch is that the practitioner's attention stays at the tip of her fingers: only with her attention there can she assess the balance of energy and structure in her client. But there is another thing too. When your attention slides away you lose awareness of the boundary between you and the object you are touching. Similarly, if your attention slides away from your fingertip when you are touching a person, you start to blend with them. So the way to maintain the boundary between you is simple: just keep your attention on it. 'Maintaining the boundary' can sound as if you need some esoteric skill or magical power in order to do it. Not at all. All you have to do is put your attention on it.

As you will see, there is a lot more to be said and understood about this focusing of attention. The unpleasant experience of being 'prodded' by another person, for example, can be explained by the fact that the other person's attention isn't on the touch itself, but is occupied with some other thought or sensation. For now I want to sum up the first aspect of interface touch: it is touching with attention at the precise location of the touch.

touching structure

The next essential quality is that the touch must be bone to bone; that is, the practitioner's bone must be in touch with the client's bone. Of course, all bones are covered by soft tissue, so it is not literally a bone contact. However, the sensation is unmistakable.

First, try pressing, with a fingertip, into an area of your body where the bone is so deeply buried in soft tissue that you cannot feel it – for example the back of the thigh. Stop pressing in when you feel it would be uncomfortable to go any further, hold the finger still for a moment or two, and notice the sensation under your fingertip. For me, it feels like a kind of diffused, tense, resistance; the resilience of the tissue is equal to the pressure of my finger, and seems to spread out all around it, fading away the further it gets from the finger. In addition, the contact is rather blurred – I do not get a precise sensation of the shape of the muscle of my thigh or of my fingertip.

Now, in contrast, try pressing your fingertip onto an area of the body where the bone is close to the surface – say on a finger or on your shin (just on the inside of your leg is best). Do it quite deliberately – don't just leave your fingertip vaguely resting on the surface. Again, only go as far as feels comfortable, and again hold the pressure for a moment or two and register the sensation.

It does feel different. Your fingertip comes to a pretty sudden stop and, as you hold the contact, you lose awareness of the soft tissue covering both the bone in your finger and the bone of your shin. You get the sensation of one bone touching another. In addition, there is a good deal of clarity about the contact; your attention seems to focus naturally on the precise area you are touching, and no other. Now try it again (if you used your shin, try your finger instead this time – and vice versa) and compare the two. With the help of the contrast, you realize that with this touch you can also discover something about the underlying bone. For me, the bone of my finger felt smooth, round and solid. The shin bone felt pitted, almost like a honeycomb, flat, and with more tension in it. Your experience of these two bones may not have been the same as mine – but I imagine that they felt different in some way.

Although these examples are of bone which is close to the skin, you can touch almost all the bones of the body – at least at some point – in this way. So with this kind of touch, you can touch the whole skeleton. Or, to use the language of Zero Balancing, you can touch structure.

touching energy

Clearly, the next step is to be able to touch energy. It is true, but not very helpful, to say as follows: given that energy flows through bone, whenever you touch bone you are bound to be touching energy, too. But, as we've just seen, there is all the difference in the world between touching something without knowing you are touching it, and touching something with awareness of what you are touching. So try the following experiment.

Grasp one forearm firmly, with the palm of your grasping hand flat on the top of the forearm. Your fingers should be wrapped round the outside of the arm and your thumb should be lying along the inside of the bone pointing straight up at your elbow. The little finger of the grasping hand should be an inch or two above the wrist. Now simultaneously pull back with your little finger and push with your thumb – as if you were trying to bend the bone in the middle – and hold it like that for about five seconds. Notice how your arm feels and then release the grasp. Most people get the feeling that the bone is bending. (If it didn't, try doing it on the other forearm. Sometimes it is clearer on one side than the other.) Of course it isn't actually bending – or, as I would prefer to put it, the structure isn't bending. But the energy is. What you are feeling is a bending of the energy flow down the bone.

There's more to say about this business of touching energy, but before I come to it I need to widen the discussion a bit. Maybe you felt something when you 'bent' your arm; if so, how do you know that it is the energy I was talking about? Maybe you didn't feel anything when you 'bent' the arm; if so, how do you know that there is anything to feel? This raises the whole puzzling business of validating any knowledge about something so...well, I almost wrote 'intangible' – and that's the problem, of course. Some people say that energy is tangible, but if you can't touch it yourself, how do you know what they're talking about, or even whether to believe them?

The first step is to realize that there is a general difficulty which applies as much to something as obvious as a car or a dog as it does to energy. If I talk to you about a dog, you summon up in your mind some image of a dog. It may not look quite like the one I'm talking about, but the word means something to you because you have had an experience of a real dog. Now imagine I use the word dog and you've never seen a real dog. I could describe one to you in endless detail, but you wouldn't be able to call up any image to make sense of what I was saying. Actually, you wouldn't really know what I was talking about. You might take it on trust that there was such a thing, somewhat like a small horse, but the word 'dog' wouldn't have any meaning for you because you have no experience of that to which the word refers.

Now substitute the phrase 'energy in the bone' for the word 'dog' – and it's pretty obvious what the problem is. Until you've had the experience of bone energy, you can't actually know what I'm talking about. But if you have had the experience of feeling bone energy, often enough to trust what you're feeling, you know exactly what I'm talking about.

How to get over this huge gap? In the case of a dog it would be easy – I'd go and find one and show it you, but I can't do that with energy in the bone. What I can suggest is that you follow the path by which all knowledge – from the most technically scientific to the most abstractly spiritual – is validated and communicated. There are three steps:

1. Do this.
2. Notice what happens.
3. Check what you noticed with others who have done these two steps.

So, for example, if you want to know if a cell really does have a nucleus, then:

1. Get a microscope, learn to take histological sections, stain the cell, put it under the microscope and look.
2. Notice what you see and describe it as accurately as you can.
3. Find a group of people who have all done exactly as you have done and compare notes. If you are all in agreement about what you saw at stage 2, then that is knowledge as reliable as any you'll ever get.

It is easy to underestimate the first step. 'Do this' can be the most creative, exciting, mind-boggling doorway to an unknown world. 'Do this' is always a method – and a really good method reveals information which is new to you and reliable too. Sometimes, it takes years of 'doing this' before you notice anything at all – sometimes it happens in an instant. (There are reasons for this, but to go into them would take us too far away from the focus of this book. Those who are interested are referred to Ken Wilber, *Sex, Ecology, Spirituality*, pp. 268–276, from which I have taken, in an abbreviated form, the content of the 'digression' above.)

What I am suggesting is that Zero Balancing is a 'Do this'. If you do it, it will lead you to an experience of energy in the body of another person, an experience which can be validated by a large community. The exercises in this book all contain this basic set of steps: Do this. Notice. Compare what you noticed to what I noticed. If you choose to do the exercises, you may well have an experience of energy, and will understand better what I'm talking about – or you may choose to simply take it on trust. You can decide, for example, that it is something like electricity, and leave it at that.

In touching bone, and in the arm bending experiment, you were doing something without quite realizing you were doing it. You were 'taking up the slack'; that is, removing the body's inherent resilience. Again, it is easiest to explain this by way of an experiment. Take a piece of cloth at least a couple of feet long. Ideally, get someone to hold one end while you hold the other – otherwise tie one end to something solid like a table leg. Let the cloth be really loose and floppy at first, then gently pull on it until it is stretched quite tight. Hold it tight for a moment or two and then gently release the tension. Notice what you feel as the cloth tightens, and again what you feel as the tension is released. Do it a few times.

There is a point as you pull when the tension in the cloth puts you in touch with the nature of what is holding it at the other end. And a point, as you slacken, when you lose that connection. This is really obvious if someone is holding the other end, but even with an inanimate object you suddenly feel linked to it. It is by taking up the slack in the cloth that you are put in touch with what is at the other end.

There is a good deal of slack in the human body. Again, try an experiment. Lie your right forearm on your lap and grasp your right wrist in your left hand. Now pull on the whole right arm across your body to the point where you can feel that your upper body wants to start to turn to relieve the tension building up in your right shoulder. Don't let it turn; keep it facing straight ahead. Now pull the right arm just a little more, again keeping your upper body in the same position, and hold the stretch for a few moments. Don't forget to breathe! Notice what you are feeling, then let go of the stretch.

What you have done is to take up the slack in the arm. Basically, there are gaps between the joints – in the wrist joint where the bones of the hand meet the bones of the arm, in the elbow joint where the bones of the forearm meet the bone of the upper arm, and in the shoulder joint where the bone of the upper arm fits into the shoulder blade. You can't pull the bones apart because there are ligaments which prevent that happening. But the ligaments aren't tight when your arm is at rest; if they were you wouldn't have the flexibility you need in your arm.

The point is that when you take up the slack in your arm you are in touch with what is at the other end, in much the same way as you were in touch with the person at the other end of the cloth once it was stretched. So what did you feel when you stretched your arm? For me, before the slack was taken up, my left hand was just touching my right hand. Once it had been taken up I felt as if that hand was touching me somewhere in my chest. In a funny sort of a way the arm disappeared. I was aware that it was tense, but not aware of it as an arm: it was like a cable through which something flowed, but it didn't have a personality, so to speak, of its own. It was the same with the cloth. Before I took up the slack, my hand was aware of the cloth, but after I had done so, I lost that and became aware of what was holding the cloth at the other end. In terms of Zero Balancing, what you are in contact with – at the other end of the cloth or of your arm – is energy. Specifically, the energy of whatever is at the other end. It is much easier to feel that if there is another person at the other end. But you can still get something of the experience with your own arm, or even with a table.

The point of all this, and it is a big one, is that in Zero Balancing the practitioner makes contact with the client's energy body only when she has taken up the slack. Once the structure is held in a state of tension, the energy body is palpable. In fact, most of the asanas, or poses, of Yoga work in exactly this way. Each pose puts a highly specific tension through the structure, which takes up the slack, and that enables contact with a particular energy flow. The tension may be small or large – I'll come later to how you know how much tension to use – but without it, most people cannot touch energy.

In fact, there are three aspects of taking up the slack. With most bones, you have to take up the slack in the soft tissue which covers them in order to be in touch with structure at all – the inside of the shin bone is an exception; there is virtually no soft tissue over the bone. So slack in soft tissue is one kind of slack that has to be taken up. Next, as in the experiment with your arm, you can take up the slack in a series of joints – cumulatively, there is quite a lot of slack in the wrist, elbow and shoulder joints. In the spine, to take another example, there are gaps between each of the vertebrae, so there is a lot of slack in the spine as a whole. Finally, and least obviously, there is slack when you touch almost any single bone firmly, because there is some movement in the joint at one end, at least – so as you press the bone you will feel some 'give' under your finger. Once you have come to the end of the 'give', you are in touch with the energy in that bone.

To summarize the key concept of interface touch: touch bone with bone and you're in touch with structure; take up the slack, in the soft tissue or the joints, and you are in touch with energy at the same time. That makes the touch very powerful. In relation to Zero Balancing, it means that you are in a position to balance a client's energy and structure. With your attention on your fingertips, you don't add to, or take away anything from, the client's own energy. That makes it safe. There is no danger of confusion between your energy and theirs. And, at least as important, it feels safe to the client. They know instinctively if your touch preserves the boundary. It is a matter of integrity – in both senses of the word. There is an honesty about the touch which is not conveying any hidden message. And, respecting the boundary of the client's body, it leaves that body in, as the dictionary defines integrity, 'an unbroken state'.

. . . .

donkey

Interface is one half of the story of touch in Zero Balancing; the other half concerns the nature of the connection made between the two people involved.

Apparently, when two donkeys walk together up a mountain path, they lean into each other as they walk. I don't actually know why they do this – after all, only a donkey could tell me – but it is reasonable to suppose that the donkey on the outside of the path feels a lot safer that way. He is leaning away from the edge, so if he slipped, or a bit of the path crumbled away as he trod on it, he would fall inwards rather than outwards. And as he is also supported by the other donkey as he walks, he might not fall at all.

It is easy to imagine that this feels very reassuring.

I wrote 'apparently' at the start of the last paragraph because I have never seen donkeys doing this. However, the day before I sat down to write this section, I was walking on a remote fell in the Lake District when I came across a donkey – the first time I had ever seen one in 30 years of tramping over those hills. So I thought I'd try it, as best I could. After leaving a suitable amount of time for introductions, I started to put my weight against the donkey. And he actually did; he leant into me as I

50

leant into him. We leant there for a while – it felt very comfortable – until he signalled, with a shake, that he'd had enough and wandered off.

The relevance of all this is that we humans act like donkeys too – we like to be supported, to lean against something. But we do have to trust what we're leaning against. This is true emotionally as well as physically. We do not care to depend on someone, emotionally, unless we trust them to support us – for it is extremely painful to do so and be let down. So, on the one hand we are very cautious about letting go and relying on someone else to hold us up – but we love it when we feel able to do so, and it is indeed safe. All this applies just as much to being touched. If we feel safe enough to yield and surrender to the touch, it feels wonderful.

In everyday life, there seem to be two ways in which we develop trust. Most often it takes time; if placing a little bit of trust in another person turns out well, you're willing to trust that person a bit more next time, and so on. Alternatively, sometimes you just trust a person immediately, instinctively. It isn't rational, because you can't explain your reasons by reference to past experience. But there is a part of you which feels safe, and is willing to trust. In the language of Zero Balancing this part of you is called your 'donkey'. And a touch which evokes that donkey, and makes it feel safe and supported, can be truly therapeutic. If the donkey part of the person feels a touch which he or she knows immediately and instinctively, is trustworthy, he or she can 'lean' on it. I'll come in a moment to the reasons why this can be so healing, but first I want to set out the qualities of a touch that enable the person who is touched to lean into it.

The first quality is that the touch has inherent mutuality. As the donkeys walk up the path, it isn't that one donkey is doing something to the other; it is more that there is a mutual accommodation to what feels comfortable to both of them. In fact, they balance each other. What is crucial about a balancing touch is that the client feels and knows – again instinctively – that the practitioner isn't doing something to them through touch: 'doing something' in the sense of imposing on them a new pattern in their structure or energy; or imposing a view of how they should be. Knowing instinctively that there is no interference of this kind going on, it is much easier for the client to trust the touch and trust the process of the therapy.

The second quality which enables the client to trust the touch is that it recognizes, and affirms, the client's individuality. The two donkeys walking up the path will be different in all sorts of ways – one may be heavier than the other, have longer legs, be more skittish and so on. What each donkey does, we may suppose, is to register the needs of the other and find some way of accommodating them in the mutual leaning. So too, each person's 'donkey' will be different. One may like to have a really firm solid touch to lean against, another may find that overwhelming; one may throw himself into the lean enthusiastically, another may be a little shy and want to edge his way into it; one may like a brisk walk, another an ambling pace. These and many other differences stem from a complex brew of those things we call personality, temperament, the psyche, personal history and so on. The point is that each of us has a donkey which is utterly individual and unique; of which we are usually not conscious at all. We can think of our donkey responding instinctively to all sorts of situations, not just to touch: some donkeys feel most comfortable in large groups, others only with one or two close friends; some donkeys like small dark old houses, others new bright ones. In relation to touch, receiving the kind of touch which your donkey likes is a bit like being in a favourite place with your favourite people. It feels very safe and very nourishing – and it does so for the deep reason that it is precisely right for you. You can lean on this touch because it recognizes who you are, and is willing to accept who you are, as you are. Again, the donkey is willing to trust because it feels that it is not being forced to be other than it is.

This is in huge contrast to so many forms of medicine and therapy. Certainly you go to a doctor or a therapist because you want something to be different in some way; you might even categorize that as 'there is something wrong with me'. But at a deeper level you feel that your complaint is an interruption, a distortion, of who you really are – you want to get back, so to speak, to how you were before. If the doctor or therapist simply concentrates on what is wrong, there is a danger that your donkey gets the message that there is no state of wellness to get back to – that the illness is who you are rather than what you've got.

One way of summing this up is to contrast two approaches: one which recognizes the individuality of each person with another which categorizes people by illness. If you have been diagnosed as a person with high blood pressure, or as a mild manic depressive or an asthmatic, you are being seen as one of a group of people defined by some pathology. But it may be that your high blood pressure, depression or asthma feels different, is different, from those of other people – and that you want this uniqueness to be recognized rather than ignored. You want to be seen as a human being rather than as a case, or an example, of an illness. And, in terms of touch, you want to be touched as an individual rather than as just another body.

As a practitioner, learning to make that 'donkey connection' with each client takes practice. Initially it is easy with some people, that is, with those who have donkeys similar to your own; after all, you know what will suit them. With others it can be difficult, and only with experience can you learn to adjust and find a mutual accommodation. This links to something described earlier. I talked about putting tension through the structure of the body in order to be in contact with its energy, and referred to the issue of knowing how much tension is needed. The way you know is to put in tension until you feel that your body is in a state of balance with the client's – or, to use the language we now know, until you feel a donkey connection between the two of you. A connection based on a mutual leaning; one where you can feel a comfortable balance between the client's structure and energy, and your own. Again, that only comes with practice. The only rule, really, is not to have expectations. Some small, delicate people, have a donkey which likes to balance against a strong tension – and the donkeys of some very large and heavy people are gentle and reticent.

It is worth adding that it is practically impossible to make that donkey connection without an interface touch. A person's donkey recognizes immediately when a practitioner is paying attention to the touch, and is reassured by that. And the donkey knows when a connection has been made with energy and structure simultaneously, and recognizes that this touches a reality of who the person is, as an individual.

Of course, all this is to provide words and explanations for what is, in the moment, a body-felt sensation and an instinctive response. What the client knows, all the client knows, is that it feels good and it feels safe. In those circumstances, there is an opening to change and to new possibilities. There is the prospect of re-organizing structure and energy in such a way as to ease pain and allow well-being in its place.

technique

. . . .

From approximately 600 hours of recording under many circumstances, we discovered that each person has a unique, predictable and recurring field characterized by such measures as colour, the quantity of the energy, the dominance of particular body areas and the completeness of the spectrum pattern. There were also individual differences in the complex dynamics or flux of the field... We discovered by recording brain waves, blood pressure changes, galvanic skin responses, heartbeat and muscle contraction simultaneously with auric changes, that changes occurred in the field before any of the other systems changed. (Valerie V. Hunt, *Infinite Mind*, p. 33)

Technique is a rather unexciting word. It suggests a routine skill, carried out in a mechanical and unthinking way. But a good technique isn't like that at all. Apart from anything else, a good technique can be refined endlessly, and it will allow more and more subtle responses to what a situation demands. Those who practise Yoga or T'ai Chi, for example, know the value of doing the basic movements and poses they learned as beginners, but with a heightened awareness of their effects. Practising and refining technique can open a door to something deeper. Again, with Yoga and T'ai Chi, only if the body possesses certain properties and characteristics can the techniques work; so practising the techniques and feeling their effect gives insight into some key aspects of the body. This is what I was referring to in Chapter 2, when I said that an instruction to 'Do this' can be a doorway into an unknown world.

Before describing the basic technique of Zero Balancing, I want to explain what that technique does; to set out the reason why it is so effective.

clearer, stronger force fields

The concept of a force field is used to explain phenomena such as the way iron filings fall into a pattern when a magnet is brought near enough to them. The magnet exerts a force field which affects the iron filings. It is all a bit abstract, but the basic idea is that it is a region of space within which a particular force – in this example, an electro-magnetic force – will have an effect and can be detected. Since the pioneering work of Robert Becker, it is abundantly clear that there is a force field in bone. That is, inside and around bone is an area within which specific and measurable forces operate; and this force also flows through and around the joints between bones. Becker found that passing very weak electrical currents through a broken bone stimulated its healing quite dramatically.

Where a joint is not working smoothly or a bone seems not to have healed, it is easy to imagine that its force field has become disturbed or distorted in some way. This is what seems to have happened to the woman I mentioned in Chapter 1, whose broken arm had healed structurally but still didn't work properly. So one way to restore normal functioning is to restore the normal, pre-existing, force field. As Valerie Hunt says in the quotation at the head of this chapter, 'changes occurred in the field before any of the other systems changed.' And the way to change the field, the basic method, is to override a disturbed or distorted force field with a clearer, stronger one.

The basic idea is simple. When you have a blocked drain, you push some sort of a rod through the blockage, or with a kitchen sink, you might use a suction plunger to free it, or some chemical which dissolves the blockage. Whichever method you use, what you are doing is introducing a new force, one stronger than the old force which is holding the blockage in place. To extend the word force to 'force field' is simply a recognition that what is actually involved is not one force but a pattern of forces; like the pattern of forces which a magnet exerts through a tray of iron filings.

So much for a 'stronger' force field, what about a 'clearer' one? That is a field which is simpler than the one it replaces. Take the analogy of ironing a creased shirt. The heat of the iron and your weight behind it will override the force field holding the material increases, and leave it in the simpler, smooth state. In the example quoted below (don't worry about the technical terms) the punchline is in the last sentence.

> Collagen fibres [which form the basic structure of bone] are formed from long sticks, like uncooked spaghetti, of a precursor molecule called tropocollagen. This compound, much used in biological research, is extracted from formed collagen...and made into a solution. A slight change in the pH of the solution then precipitates collagen fibres. But the fibres thus formed are a jumbled, felt like mass, nothing like the layered parallel strands of bone. However, when we passed a very weak direct current through the solution, the fibres formed in rows perpendicular to the lines of force... (Robert O. Becker and Gary Selden, *The Body Electric*, p. 129)

The 'very weak direct current' which turned the jumbled mass into layered parallel strands can be seen as a clearer, stronger force field. Again, the 'clearer field' is one which simplifies the previous field. So, to take a rather different example, if you have a complex and difficult problem and you have a good talk with a friend which clarifies it, what has happened is that it all seems simpler. You realize what is really important and what is not, what needs to be done soon and what can be put off, and what you really want out of the situation. Generalizing from all this, it seems that when our bodies or our minds are disturbed, healing involves replacing that disturbance with simplicity.

Zero Balancing works by putting a clearer, stronger force field through any part of the skeleton where structure and energy are not in balance. There is one basic technique which does this.

the fulcrum

In mechanics, a fulcrum is a prop on which a lever is balanced; for example, the support in the middle of a see-saw. This prop, not very interesting at first sight, appears to be sitting there doing nothing. But think of the phrase 'Give me a fulcrum and I will move the world', and it looks a bit different. If you've ever tried to shift a big rock with a crowbar, or lever open a door, you'll know that putting a fulcrum underneath the crowbar multiplies the power you have available out of all recognition. With the fulcrum, there is a possibility of movement where there was none before. The same is true of the humble see-saw. A plank resting on the ground offers limited scope for play. Lift it on a fulcrum, and all sorts of balancing games become possible.

Zero Balancing works by placing fulcrums on the body. By using touch, it creates still points on which the body can balance. The brilliance of this idea is precisely that a fulcrum doesn't do anything itself; it just creates possibilities. A whole therapy based on not doing anything! And yet it's such an extraordinary and elegant solution to so many problems.

So the practitioner doesn't do anything to the client; what's so smart about that? For one thing it is awfully safe. The first rule of medicine is 'Do no harm'. This rule is built into the whole idea of a fulcrum; the most fundamental technique of Zero Balancing. It is there in everything the practitioner does. For another thing, highly unusual if not unique in therapies and forms of medicine which work on the body, the client is in charge of what happens. Not necessarily consciously or deliberately, but if something happens, if something changes, as a result of a fulcrum, then it has to be that the client – somehow or other – allowed that change. In other words – again an enormous statement in the context of any therapeutic system – this therapy recognizes that the client knows better than the therapist. It is the client who knows when, and how, and how much, and where to change. The therapist just puts in the fulcrum and waits; waits to see what use, if any, the client wants to make of it. This is a therapy which is a manifestation of the ancient wisdom of Lao Tzu, and gives meaning to his apparent paradoxes: 'The Master does nothing, yet he leaves nothing undone', and 'When his work is done, the people say, "Amazing: we did it, all by ourselves!"' (Stephen Mitchell (tr.), *Tao Te Ching*, nos 38 & 17).

There are a number of ways of attempting to answer the question, why it works. I could say it works because the fulcrum establishes a clearer, stronger force field – and that is true. I could say that it provides an opportunity for the body to re-organize around the point of the fulcrum – and that is true, too. But these words are really only attempts to satisfy that part of our mind which wants explanations for everything. Really, it is a mystery. And there are times when it seems better to celebrate the mystery rather than to try to explain it. It works.

There are two ways of putting in a fulcrum. One is by direct touch onto bone. For example, with the client lying on his back, the practitioner folds her hand under the back and feels the bone of a rib under one or more fingertips. From her training and through experience, she can recognize a quality in the bone which tells her whether a fulcrum is needed and if so exactly where it should be placed. Then, lifting the fingers with their natural curve, she touches the rib at interface and makes a donkey connection with the client. Then she adds a little more lift, and holds the fingers still for a few moments. That is the fulcrum – and it creates a clearer, stronger force field. Often she will then feel movement under her fingers – it is rather like touching a hose pipe when someone turns on the tap or feeling an ice cream melt on the tongue. To use the explanation in the previous paragraph, the practitioner feels the body reorganizing around the still point. (The term 'still point' doesn't have a technical meaning here, as it does in cranio-sacral therapy.)

The curve of the fingers is interesting and important. It doesn't come from the shoulder or the arm or even the hand itself, which is lying, back down, on the couch. It is just what happens naturally if you lift the fingers alone; they curve towards the wrist. The curve of the rib is met by a curve in the hand; as we will see, it is a principle of Zero Balancing that the work matches the natural curvatures in the skeleton. Intriguingly, C.P.E. Bach, writing of his even more famous father, Johann Sebastian Bach, said that, 'he played with curved fingers with the tips perpendicular to the keys and with a very quiet hand and arm' (William A. Palmer (ed.),

J.S Bach, p. 7). Substitute the word 'bone' for the word 'keys' and it is a perfect description of how to put in a fulcrum. Perhaps it is simply a perfect description of how to create a still point – in the body or in music – through touch.

The other way of creating a fulcrum is through traction. One example is a fulcrum on the neck. Sitting close to the crown of the client's head, the practitioner picks up the head, again with curved fingers on bone, and by lifting the fingers with their natural curve, pulls it gently upwards and towards her. Having taken up the slack, she adds a little more traction and holds the head in that position for a few moments. This creates the fulcrum; the still point at which the energy and structure of the neck are engaged and around which they can re-organize. In Zero Balancing, this basic fulcrum with traction, used in other parts of the body too, is called a half moon vector – or half moon for short.

It is easier to see the first kind of fulcrum I mentioned as a fulcrum; fingertips on a rib really do resemble the fulcrum of a see-saw. With this second kind, the fulcrum isn't at the same place as the fingertips; it is created by the traction, and exists somewhere in the neck between the fingertips at one end and those vertebrae lower down the spine which do not move significantly as a result of the traction. One of the many skills of the practitioner is to know where that fulcrum needs to be placed and how much traction is needed to create it there. It is helpful, with this kind of fulcrum, to think of it less as a point and more as the establishment of a clearer, stronger force field which will be stronger and more focused in one particular place, but which has a widespread effect.

There are many variations on these two basic fulcrums. Here are two examples, just to give an idea of the richness of the concept and the way it can be developed in order to touch structure and energy at particular places on the body. First, consider the large movements of the neck. It can flex down to the chest and extend to lift the face to the sky; it can rotate to left or right; and it can bend to cock the head sideways. Now the basic half moon on the neck, described above, will clearly have an effect in the ability of the neck to flex and extend – both the traction and the curve are along that axis. But it doesn't relate to the two other movements. If the practitioner wants to affect either or both of these, a simple variation of the basic fulcrum will do the trick. As she puts in the basic fulcrum, she starts to add in a twist, which will involve an element of rotation and side bending. Holding the fulcrum for a few moments, a clearer, stronger force field is being put through all three main movements of the neck. This has a powerful effect, and the resulting improvement in mobility of the neck is often dramatic.

The other example I want to give here is one which combines both kinds of fulcrum, touching bone and traction. Standing opposite the soles of the client's feet, the practitioner picks up the foot by interlinking her fingers on the top and letting her thumbs rest lightly on the sole. Thus her fingers rest directly on the tarsal joints of the foot. Now she applies traction which engages the energy body, and then lifts her fingers upwards and towards her with a curved movement. This half moon, created by the direct pressure of her fingers on the tarsal joints, is again a very powerful fulcrum.

Claiming that a fulcrum is powerful is based not on some notion of what it should do, but on direct observation of its effects. Certainly, some of the outcomes of a fulcrum, or a session as a whole, may not be felt for some time – there is more on this in later chapters. But built into the format of a Zero Balancing session is the practice of evaluation and re·evaluation. It is a very straightforward practice. Before the practitioner puts in a fulcrum, she evaluates. In the case of a joint, she moves it gently through its normal range of motion. So with the foot, for example, she will press up against the ball of the foot until it is flexed and then release the pressure – simulating the movement of the foot when walking. She will register, mainly with her hands but also with her eyes, the quality and quantity of movement. Does it move freely, or are there jerky discontinuities? Does it come to a sudden stop or gradually slow as tension builds in the ligaments? Does the foot splay out or swing back in a straight arc? These are some of the observations she will make. She then has a clear benchmark for any work she may do. After she has put a fulcrum into the foot she can re-evaluate its movement and see if there is any improvement. If there is, the fulcrum has done its job.

Put like this, it all sounds quite commonplace. But I will never forget the chiropractor who, at his first Zero Balancing workshop, evaluated the movement of my right foot, which had been causing me some problems ever since I'd carried some very heavy luggage a few weeks before. From his wrinkled forehead, I could see him thinking, 'Hmmm, there is a real problem here; needs a good deal of manipulation...now how would I go about that? Not easy...' As he evaluated he was lost in thought, so I suggested that he try putting in a foot fulcrum; his first. Bringing himself back to the workshop, he did so and stood back. 'Now re-evaluate', I reminded him. I can still see the look of astonishment on his face. He just couldn't believe the change that had taken place. It blew away his assumption, that only by manipulation could such a change be brought about.

So the practice of evaluating and re-evaluating is a key part of putting in a fulcrum; apart from anything else, it tells you when you have done enough. As artists (and writers) learn, the great skill is in knowing when to stop. But there is more to it than that. Of course, a practitioner can put in a fulcrum, re-evaluate, and find no change, or an insignificant change. She might try again – maybe the fulcrum wasn't placed very precisely; maybe she didn't really make a connection with the client's donkey; maybe she didn't hold it quite long enough. But if there is still no change after a second try, she will leave it and move on. After all, she knows that the purpose of a fulcrum is not to force change on a client but to create an opportunity for change if that is appropriate. Beyond all that however, the discipline of evaluating and re-evaluating keeps the practitioner real and grounded and honest. It is all too easy, with many therapies and systems of medicine, to argue, 'Well it ought to be working, so I'll assume it is working.' The fact is, if you re-evaluate and nothing has changed, then nothing has changed. It doesn't mean you were wrong to try; but it does mean you don't kid yourself.

I said earlier that the full effects of a fulcrum may not be felt for some time; maybe later during the session, maybe hours, days, or weeks afterwards. There are a host of reasons for this. It may take time for other parts of the body to respond to the change at that place; it may take the client time to realize, for example, that he is dealing better with the stresses of his life, and so on. But for all that, the test of re-evaluation is a very good one. If there is a big change in movement, then there has been a big change in the energy and structure of that joint, and this will have a beneficial effect on the body, mind or spirit, or some combination of all three.

To sum up this chapter: the method of Zero Balancing is to put a clearer, stronger force field through the skeleton. And that clearer, stronger field is created by the technique of a fulcrum whose effectiveness is tested by the practice of evaluation and re-evaluation. The next chapter looks at the key places on the body where a fulcrum will have the most effect, and also at the kinds of effect it may have.

the body

· ·

Without warning, the patient sat up in bed and shouted.

"I see everything twice!"

A nurse screamed and an orderly fainted.

Doctors came running from every direction with needles, tubes, rubber mallets and oscillating metal tines... A colonel with a large forehead and horn rimmed glasses soon arrived at a diagnosis.

"It's meningitis," he called out emphatically, waving the others back...

"...why pick meningitis?" inquired a major with a suave chuckle. "Why not, let's say, acute nephritis?"

"Because I'm a meningitis man, that's why, and not an acute nephritis man," retorted the colonel. (Joseph Heller, *Catch 22*, pp. 192–193)

All forms of medicine and healing take a perspective on the organization and functioning of the human body. All have a set of ideas and assumptions which seek to account for the way it is, and as a consequence the way it could change. This is mainly because of the enormous complexity of the body; any practitioner has to use some simplifying device to select what is noticed and what is of interest. An osteopath notices the relationships of bones, ligaments and tendons precisely because her skill lies in adjusting those relationships. A doctor tends to notice deviations from the chemical norms of the body, because chemical drugs are his main form of intervention. And behind both of these lies a deeper perception of the nature and workings of the human body.

William Harvey's discovery of the circulation of the blood stemmed from his perception of the heart as a pump. This seems commonplace now, but it was remarkable at the time and one with dramatic and far-reaching consequences. For one thing, this perception had enormous explanatory power. It explained the pulsing in the wrists, neck and ankles, and the surges of blood from a severed artery. It explained how nutrients were dispersed through the body and why a person dies when the heart stops beating, and much, much more. So it suggested a host of remedies for a host of illnesses and complaints. The benefits were, and are, enormous. But it ignored a lot too.

For one thing, the perception of the heart as a pump carries an implicit assumption that it is machine-like. So if the heart is not working well – say one of the valves is not closing quite as firmly as it should – then the obvious implication is that it needs to be fixed in the way you would fix a leaky valve in a machine. What this leaves out of the picture is thousands of years of human perception that the heart is somehow the residence of love in the body. Even without the romantic stuff, phrases like 'my heart went out to him' or 'heartfelt thanks' bear witness to this continuous perception. So, from this perspective, if the heart is not working well, it may have something to do with 'heartbreak' or 'heartache'.

Now this is not to say that it is a bad idea to replace a defective valve. It is just a reminder that any perception of the body has its bias, and Western medicine, in general, is biased towards seeing the body as a machine; sometimes a mechanical machine, sometimes a chemical machine. The perception of the body which colours Zero Balancing is that of an inter-related structure and energy. This raises the question, 'What aspect of the body is highlighted by this perception, and what kind of benefits might flow from treatments based on it?' The rest of this chapter seeks to answer these questions.

foundation joints

In the first chapter I said that Zero Balancing sees the whole skeleton as one functional unit, but that doesn't mean that the practitioner has to work on every bone and every joint. By working mainly on a particular set of joints, touching bone there, she can balance energy and structure in the whole structure.

To describe these joints, and to explain why work on them can affect the whole, it helps to distinguish between joints which are freely movable and those which are not. Some joints, the freely movable ones, are spanned by muscles which can be specifically activated. Accordingly, you can move the bone on one side of the joint by a deliberate act of will. You can choose to lift your lower arm or your leg, so your elbow joint and your knee joint are freely movable. By contrast, there are many joints we can't move – we don't realize this because we never have to think about moving them. To be crystal clear, there is movement in these joints, which results from forces acting on that joint, but it is not a movement you can initiate or control. The term 'foundation joints' refers to these kinds of joints. There is also a further category of joints, called 'semi-foundation joints', which have the same general properties as foundation joints, but have a slightly greater degree of movement.

The effects of working on foundation and semi-foundation joints can be dramatic. Very early on in my training, I gave a session to a middle-aged Yoga teacher who was having a problem with one of her hips. Before starting, I asked the normal safety questions about her medical history and she told me that her right shoulder had been injured in a bomb blast in the Second World War. 'Since then I have been able to move that arm backwards and forwards, but I can't lift it at all', she told me. I did the session, not touching her shoulder or arm – there was no point. She came back a week or so later and I asked how her hip was. 'Well, it's a bit better, not much', she said. 'But look at this.' And as she spoke, she lifted her right arm in a full flowing movement. I couldn't believe it and neither could she. What I didn't know then, and know now, is that creating a clear flow of energy through foundation joints can have widespread and powerful effects.

There is a complex set of joints in both hands and feet which are not freely movable, and which are foundation joints. You can move your fingers and toes, and your wrist and ankle – but between the fingers and the wrist, and between the toes and the ankle is a set of bones which you cannot move (Figures 6 (a) and 6 (b)). In fact, looking at this figure, the similarity of structure is very obvious. It appears we need this set of small bones even though we can't, so to speak, do anything with them. Looking at the cross section along the foot, Figure 7 (a), you can see that the five bones (shaded in the drawing) form the keystone of the arch of the foot. For simplicity, I am going to refer to all five together as one foundation joint. Look, too, at the cross section across the foot, Figure 7 (b), and you will notice that these same bones form another arch.

(a)   *(b)*

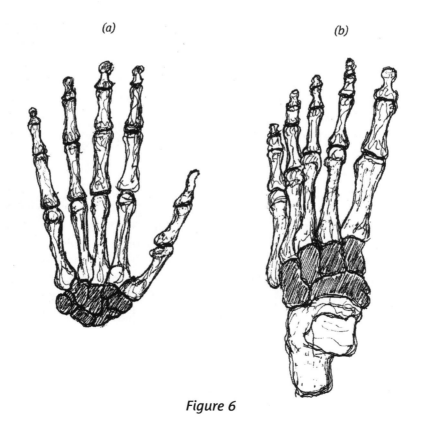

Figure 6

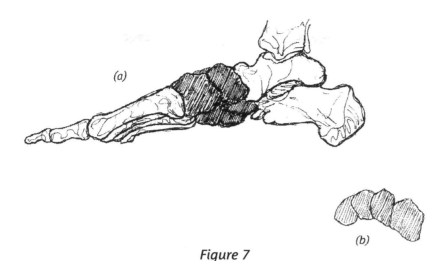

(a)

(b)

Figure 7

Just as in a bridge or a cathedral, these arches allow weight to be carried over a space. As you walk or run, the whole weight of the body comes down on the foot and if it is not to be crushed – or at least badly bruised – on impact, there must be space underneath it. The arch of the foot spreads the weight over a space so that it can be absorbed through the heel, the ball of the foot, and the toes. This absorption of the impact protects the skeleton as a whole from shock waves coming up from the foot as you land.

So this foundation joint is structurally crucial; and, as you would expect, it is energetically crucial too. In fact, all foundation joints are energetically crucial. They transmit forces in and through the body; and, in my dictionary, 'force' is a synonym for energy. One way of explaining why we cannot move these joints voluntarily is to say that as their main function is to transmit forces, it is better if we can't control these. Or we'd think we'd know how to do it better, and start mucking around with an exquisitely well-organized system!

Imagine a very strong flow of energy coming straight down the leg – think of it as a flow of water if that helps you to envisage it. As it gets to the ankle, some of it will flow straight down the heel, into the ground (Figure 8). And some of it will need to make a very sharp turn to flow along the foot and into the ground at the ball of the foot and toes. Where there is a sharp turn, the flow will speed up – think of water again. Now that fast flow has to be dispersed to flow down the five metatarsal bones – and from there to the ball of the foot at the end of the metatarsals, and to the toes. It is clear that the bones of this foundation joint will serve to break up one strong current into five weaker ones, much as large rocks will do in a river.

In addition, where there is a sharp bend in a river, you'll see a speeding up of the flow on the outside of the bend, and a back eddy being created on the inside of the bend. Applying that analogy here, you would expect to find a back eddy of energy on the top of the joint (Figure 9). This eddy will have the effect of providing a force which will lift the joint and reinforce the arch: energy and structure working together. Beautiful.

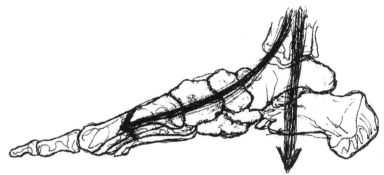

Figure 8

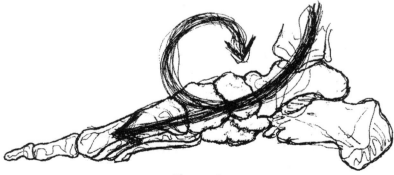

Figure 9

Now if this foundation joint is not working well, for example the five bones are misaligned, then there are three immediately obvious consequences. First, the person cannot restore the alignment by deliberately moving the bones in the joint. With a bit of luck, some accidental jarring of the foot might joggle them back into place – but much more likely is that they will stay stuck out of place for a long time. Second, the body will start to compensate for this distortion consciously, if the person is in pain, or unconsciously, if they aren't. The person will start to walk in such a way that the other parts of the foot and leg can cope as best they can with the limitations of the foundation joint. In the short term, this is a sensible strategy, but in the longer term it is likely that the adjustments will, themselves, start to cause problems – after all, none of them will hold the skeleton in its ideal form. A problem in the foot, for example, can often cause knock-on problems in the knee and even the hip joints. So not only is the initial problem likely to be long-lasting, it is also likely to have wider ramifications. Neither of these points holds true for a freely movable joint; as long as the misalignment is not too severe the person can usually joggle things back into place quite quickly by exercising the relevant muscles. Finally, there will be consequences, too, from the interruption to the ideal flow of energy through that joint. Briefly – there will be more about this in the next section – the main flow through the vertical skeleton won't connect properly with the ground, and the person may well have difficulty in 'standing up for himself' or 'standing on his own two feet' or 'standing firm': clichés of this kind usually have a basis in old wisdom.

There is a clear implication from all this. If there is a misalignment in a foundation joint, then an outside agent is normally needed to help restore normal functioning. With many therapies you might wonder if you could do the work on yourself and by yourself. But if the source of a problem is in a foundation joint, you can't. In addition, even if there is no major problem with a foundation joint, it is likely that there will be minor misalignments in at least some of them; resolving these can be seen as sensible preventive medicine, ensuring that the joints are restored to their proper functioning before any widespread compensations set in. And the effects of working on a foundation joint will not only bring benefits to other places in the skeleton but also to what is normally regarded as quite separate from the skeleton – a person's mental or emotional disposition.

I say more about this idea in the next section. For now, to summarize, I simply want to point out that, given a perception of the body as inter-related energy and structure, foundation and semi-foundation joints – where structure and energy are most intimately connected – are the places where a fulcrum is likely to have the most effect.

. . . .

physical, mental and emotional

I suggested that when a clear flow of energy is re-established through the feet, a person may find it easier to 'stand up for himself' or to 'stand on his own two feet'. Similarly, it is a common turn of phrase to say that a person is 'stiff-necked'. Interestingly, similar phrases turn up in other languages – such associations are made not just by one culture or society but seem to have deeper roots than that. In other words, different areas of the body have long been associated with particular emotions, mental states, issues in life and so on. Given that Zero Balancing has such a powerful effect on the body, it is reasonable to suppose that it will have effects on the emotions, mental states and issues which are connected with the areas on which it works. It seems to be the case that bringing more balance into a particular area also brings more balance into the rather more intangible aspects of ourselves which are lodged there.

I hesitated before writing 'lodged there' at the end of the last sentence. I realize that it is quite a big step from saying that a mental state, for example, is 'associated with' or 'connected to' a particular area of the body to claiming that it is 'lodged there'. And that step challenges the view of the body which has been accepted in Western culture for the last 300 years. This view is that body and mind are separate, and that the activity of the mind takes place only in the brain, which is in the head. It is simply nonsense, in this view, to suggest that a mental state might be lodged in the foot.

In the past 300 years science and its methods have been extraordinarily successful and they have been applied – also with remarkable success – to illness and disease. There is no doubt about the value of trying to find a cause and effect relationship between, for example, stress and debilitation of the immune system, as a way of seeking to explain why it is that when people are stressed they tend to fall ill more easily and recover more slowly. But we all know that when people are stressed they do, in fact, get ill more easily, even if we don't have an explanation for it. In other words something may be true before science has found an explanation for that truth. This point may seem too obvious to labour, but it is ignored all the time. There really is a difference between something being true and finding a scientific explanation for it. There are lots of things which are true but the scientific explanation for them just hasn't yet been found. There may well be lots of things which are true and for which no scientific explanation will ever be found – they simply won't be revealed by its methods. You cannot see an emotion through a microscope; equally, you cannot know the chemical composition of an amino acid by sheer intuition. So, although there may be no scientific proof that a mental state or an emotion is lodged in a particular part of the body, it may still be true.

The following examples describe the structure, the energy and the issues that are touched on in a Zero Balancing session, all together. I could describe all the areas of the body in a similar way, but these three examples will carry the main ideas.

the feet

Charles had a bad accident as a child when both feet were crushed and the bones re-set. His feet have given him problems ever since. They often hurt, and he walks unsteadily, very much on the outside of his feet. When you meet him, you notice two things straight away. He is very jolly, cracking endless jokes, shouting with laughter at any opportunity and including everyone within earshot in his conversation. Everything is amusing, but in a heavy kind of a way. No lightness, or real, unforced gaiety. You also can't help noticing that his upper body is very large, but his legs are like matchsticks; they took as if they've been stuck on as an afterthought. Not really functional, they're just there to make up the numbers. And indeed he has very little strength in them, and finds it difficult to walk any distance or to get out of a low chair.

On the couch, his feet come as a bit of a shock. They aren't foot shaped. Virtually square, they are almost as wide at the heel as they are at the ball of the foot and almost as deep at the toes as they are at the ankle. His toes are pulled right back so the tips are on the ground but the middle joint is high in the air. And there is practically no movement in them at all – they just don't budge when you push against the ball of the foot.

Talking to him about his life is quite distressing too. Having inherited a lot of money and a large farm, he is now practically bankrupt. He is engaged in a number of lawsuits, which have gone on for years, having refused to settle them on reasonably advantageous terms. His wife is ill and depressed at the constant threat hanging over her of losing her home and the farm, and of being poor in her old age. She is angry with him, but he tells her she worries too much, so their relationship isn't good. All this is bad enough, but more distressing is the fact that he recounts all this as a merry adventure, and intersperses the tale with his excitement at a whole series of new projects, all of which appear impractical and involve battles with various authorities.

It isn't too far-fetched to imagine that the massive restriction in his feet has made it difficult for him to move flexibly through the ups and downs of life, absorbing the shocks as he goes. Over the years, movement has become difficult – which is reflected both in the shape of his body and in the shape of his affairs. He tends to get locked into a position, and can't move away from it. He is ungrounded, and this may have contributed both to the situation he is in, and to the unrealistic ways he plans to get out of it; even to his forced joviality.

I tell Charles' story mainly as an example of the consequences which may be attributed in part to restriction in the feet, but it is worth adding that Zero Balancing is helping. After about six sessions, over a period of six months, his feet are beginning to look more normal, and he has movement in them. He has dropped some of his more hare-brained projects and seems to be applying himself to bringing the lawsuits to an end. As I write, I don't know what the outcome will be, or how much change is possible. But to his endless credit, he is persisting with the sessions even though they are bringing change to how he has been for 50 years. Charles doesn't lack courage.

the dorsal hinge

This is not a term used in conventional anatomy textbooks, but it refers to an important area: one which links two types of structure and two types of movement. The structure of the rib cage is ingeniously arranged to allow the movement required for breathing. As I mentioned in Chapter 1, on the in-breath, each rib lifts upwards and outwards and rotates around its axis, and these movements are reversed on the out-breath. At the same time the rib cage provides a strong protective enclosure for the heart and lungs. So practically no flexion (bending forward) is possible in this part of the trunk; if there were, then the rib cage might crush the very organs it serves to protect. Not much extension (bending backward) is possible either – that would open up the rib cage and leave the organs vulnerable. By far the freest movement of the upper, thoracic spine is rotation. The rib cage as a whole can swing around a central axis, so the shoulders can be facing sideways while the hips face straight ahead. Accordingly, the vertebrae of the thoracic spine are shaped to allow this kind of movement (Figure 10 (a)).

The lower, lumbar spine, by contrast, doesn't have to support the rib cage; so it is here that flexion and extension can happen. But rotation is very restricted by the way the lumbar vertebrae interlock to give stability to the spine as a whole (Figure 10 (b)).

To sum up, there has to be some ingenious link between the upper part of the spine which can rotate but not flex or extend much, and the lower part which can flex or extend but which can't rotate much. There is one vertebra which carries out this linking function. Its superior articular processes are shaped like those of a thoracic vertebra, allowing rotation, and its inferior processes are shaped like those of a lumbar vertebra, preventing rotation but allowing flexion and extension (Figure 10 (c)). You can think of this vertebra as providing a 'hinge' between the two sections of the spine – hence its name, the dorsal hinge.

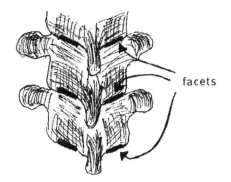

THORACIC VERTEBRAE

(a)

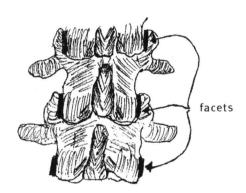

LUMBAR VERTEBRAE

(b)

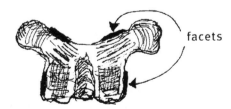

DORSAL HINGE VERTEBRAE

(c)

Figure 10

There are two reasons why the dorsal hinge is structurally so important. First, movements of the spine as a whole entail a series of small movements of individual vertebrae – each adding a little to the total range of motion. Restriction in the movement available to one vertebra will therefore make a relatively small difference to the total range, and, indeed, often a restriction in one is compensated for by increased mobility in others. But because it is unique, any restriction in the dorsal hinge vertebra will directly limit the available movement of the whole spine. And, again because it is unique, other vertebrae cannot compensate for restrictions there.

Second, the function of this vertebra is quite likely to be restricted in some way. Any movement which combines flexion and rotation in the whole spine will involve more stress on the dorsal hinge than on any other vertebra. Simple movements, such as bending to one side and lifting or looking over one's shoulder, are common everyday examples of such combined movements. In addition, as we have seen, the vertebrae of the lumbar spine don't allow rotation in that area, and the first joint below the dorsal hinge which can transmit any rotary force is the sacro-iliac joint. So if there are restrictions in the sacro-iliac joint, and there often are, they will directly affect the dorsal hinge. And vice versa. Much lower back pain comes from stress in one of these joints affecting the other; and fulcrums in both can bring quick and lasting relief.

This view of the dorsal hinge as an area of transition also finds echoes in energy anatomy described by the chakra system (Figure 11). In that system, there is a substantial and often difficult transition between the third chakra – located just above the navel – and the fourth chakra, which lies in the centre of the chest, between the breasts. The three lower chakras are essentially concerned with what makes a human being individual, unique, different from all others, whereas the upper four chakras link the individual to what is shared with all humanity; perhaps more precisely, to an experience of unity with all things. The energy of the lower three chakras helps the task of individuation which is the necessary preoccupation of the first half of life; becoming separate from the mother, the family, the tribe, the conventions of a society and so on. Having done that, it is not easy for an individual to shift his or her focus;

between the third and fourth chakras lies a change from the energies of separation to the energies of union.

It is fascinating to notice that the diaphragm, that strong muscle which divides the trunk in two so dramatically and separates the chest cavity from the abdomen, lies between the third and fourth chakras and almost always attaches to the rib which is attached to the dorsal hinge vertebra. As ever, structure and energy mirror one another.

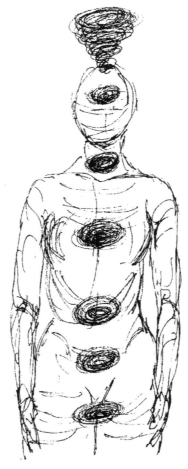

Figure 11

the shoulder girdle

With our arms we bring things towards us; food to the mouth, soap to the skin, and a loved one into an embrace. With movement in the opposite direction, we give things to others, and we push away what we don't want. We interact with the world through our arms, and the more flexibility there is here the more easily we can respond to the demands and gifts that come our way. If you try moving your arms in all directions, you'll notice that the range of what we can grasp in our hands, without moving the body, is astonishing. There are two structural features which make this possible. One is that the shoulder joint itself, where the bone of the upper arm fits into an indentation in the shoulder blade, is a ball and socket joint. This kind of joint allows full rotation – and the socket is a very shallow one, which increases the range available. That is why dislocations of the shoulder are pretty common – it doesn't take much force to push the bone out of the socket.

The other structural feature is that the collar bone and shoulder blade, which create and support the socket of the joint, are only attached to the trunk with one small semi-foundation joint. It is at the front of the body, at a spot just below the throat, about half an inch out from the mid-line. It is here that the collar bone attaches to the sternum. It is absolutely extraordinary that the arm only actually hitches onto the trunk here; you would never guess if you didn't know. So the whole assembly of collar bone and shoulder blade – the shoulder girdle – is resting on top of the rib cage, only lightly held in place, and free to move in many planes.

In fact the main restrictions to movement of the arm usually come from the way the shoulder blade rests on the rib cage: if it can move freely, so can the arm. Looking at another person's back as they move their arm up and down, across and out, shrugging their shoulders, hugging themselves, or putting their shoulders back like a soldier, you can see the shoulder blade moving over a surprising distance under the skin. None of these movements would be possible if the shoulder blade could not float on the ribs. So between rib and blade is muscle which, apart from enabling certain movements, also provides a cushion between them. And under that muscle is a bursa, a fluid-filled pad, which acts as a lubricant. The muscle and the bursa together maintain flexibility in the movements

79

of the arm as a whole, and also act as a shock absorber. A sudden force coming up the arm – imagine you are pushing on something which suddenly jams tight – is absorbed there. Or, to put it another way, if it is not absorbed there, then the shock is transmitted right into the body.

As ever, what is structural is also energetic. Instinctively, we pick up how a person interacts with the world by noticing their shoulders. Drooping shoulders express a feeling of hopelessness; the person has given up even trying to prevent the shocks of the world reaching the trunk. Stiff and tense shoulders convey a message of rigidity, even defensiveness. One way this can happen is through an emotional shock coming up the arm and being transmitted into the body. Imagine reaching out to comfort or embrace someone who is normally pleased to be touched by you, but who this time rejects the offer, and you can see how the shock of this might hit you through the shoulder. That may make the muscle and bursa compress, as a physical shock would do, which, in turn, will restrict movement in the whole shoulder girdle. This experience may then make it harder, both physically and emotionally, to reach out openly and freely in future. A hug from someone who has had a shock of this kind may feel stiff and tense.

A frozen shoulder, to take the most extreme example of problems in this area, is notoriously hard to treat. Not surprising really; clearly something has gone very wrong to create such a dramatic contrast to how the shoulder should be. What will be at issue will be some kind of disruption in the relationship between the person and his or her world. Fulcrums in the semi-foundation joint, where the collar bone joins the trunk, can certainly help. So too can fulcrums into the ribs which lie underneath the shoulder blade. But for this, and for less acute problems, there is another fulcrum which often has a remarkable effect. A fulcrum placed in the centre of the shoulder blade helps restore the physical freedom of movement, the energetic insulation and an openness to relating to others. In fact, this fulcrum is a prime example of the general point that in the stillness of a fulcrum the body will do what it needs. Who would have thought that a fulcrum which compresses the space beneath the shoulder blade could increase its effectiveness? But it does.

the whole

At the end of a Zero Balancing session, the practitioner picks up the client's feet and, applying traction with a gentle curve to the point where she is in good contact with the donkey, holds the fulcrum for a few moments to integrate all the work she has done. I want to close this chapter in the same spirit.

Every fulcrum has a curve in it somewhere. The half moon from the feet which I mentioned before, and which is used a number of times in a session, has a curve. So does the half moon vector from the head which, again, is used a number of times in a session. So do fulcrums which are simple lifting ones, on the sacro-iliac joint for example. This is because the natural shape of the fingers as they lift upwards is curved, and this curve imparts a curved force into the body. There are no straight lines on the body. So it is plain common sense to hold a curved shape in a curve – imagine holding a ball on a flat plate, and then imagine holding it in a bowl. But there is more to it than that.

The most important curves, structurally, are the curves of the spine. For one thing, they enable the body to carry vastly more weight than it could if the spine were straight. For another, they keep the centre of gravity of this complex, vertical, human body directly over the mid-point between the feet while at the same time enabling balance to be maintained when the body is in motion. If there were no curves it would topple over easily. Now, if the practitioner were to put in straight traction from the feet, its force would run through these curves, tending to flatten them out (Figure 12 (a)). This would introduce stresses between the vertebrae as they reacted to the uneven pressure placed on them, flattening one side of the discs between them and stretching the other. The force of a curved traction, by contrast will, in some places, exactly match the curve of the spine. It is easy to see that a half moon from the feet will induce a flow which follows the curves of the coccyx and sacrum, and easy to realize that this will feel good to the client. However, you can see from Figure 12 (b) that when the force of the half moon reaches the lumbar spine, it would appear not to follow the convex curve of the spine, but to be its mirror image, to be concave instead. So it would appear: but it doesn't work like that. And to understand why, we come back again to the basic ideas of fulcrums and donkeys.

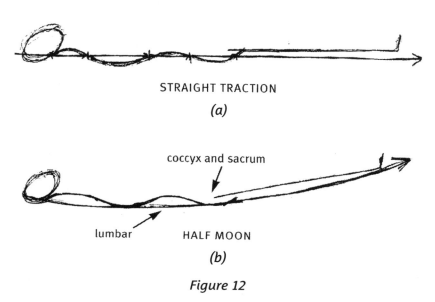

STRAIGHT TRACTION

(a)

HALF MOON

(b)

Figure 12

Think of the half moon not as an imposition on the client, but as an offering. 'I have a suggestion', the practitioner can be thought of as saying. 'Here is a new force field, very like the one you already have, but which may feel fresher, a little rejuvenated. Would you prefer this one to the old?' Putting such a question to the client's donkey, framed in a way so that it can respond naturally – that's the curve again – makes all the difference. It means that the body can take up the offering and make it its own. The half moon from the feet flows along all the curves of the spine, whether they are concave or convex because, and only if, the body accepts it and makes its own use of it. That is the beauty of Zero Balancing. And the skill of the practitioner, which can be honed endlessly, is to know, through touch, how to make that suggestion, how to ask that question in such a way as to allow the body to respond naturally, gratefully and with a sense of relief. Relief that behind all the facades, all the resistances, and all the efforts to keep up appearances, it feels truly recognized and respected.

the session

· ·

As I walked around I felt as if my body had been newly aligned in a way that it hadn't been for a very long time, perhaps since I'd started to walk. Everything seemed to be in its place, balanced with one bit on top of another just as it was meant to be. It was a lovely feeling, as if my head was connected to the sky and being gently pulled up with a string, my middle was stretched so there was lots of room for breathing and for the expansion of all the internal organs, and my legs, through the feet, were really firmly in touch with the ground. (Myra Connell, private communication)

People come for Zero Balancing for a very wide variety of reasons. Those who have never been before usually have a specific symptom like a bad back or a stiff neck, although as appreciation of the nature of complementary therapies grows, more and more are coming because, 'I am stressed' or, 'I don't feel right in myself.' Frequently, as with any therapy, once the practitioner starts to enquire about the initial reason for coming, a further and deeper reason is revealed. Many new clients have seen the effects of the work on family or friends and say to themselves (in the immortal words of the woman at the restaurant in the film *When Harry met Sally*), 'I'll have whatever she's having.' In these kinds of cases, what they are referring to is not usually some relief from symptoms but an air of well-being, of standing taller, in all senses of the phrase, and being more present.

Some of this holds true for clients who have had a number of sessions. They too will return when they have a specific problem, or they may have a condition – such as an elderly man with stiffening hips – which is kept within acceptable limits by having Zero Balancing every few months. But most of them tend to come when they know they need a session – and they know it because they recognize the difference between how they felt in the weeks immediately after their last one, and how they feel now. One client of mine comes very irregularly. I may see her three times in as many weeks and then not for months on end. The signal that finally gets her to phone for an appointment is when she has lost what she calls her 'flexibility' in dealing with her work and relationships. Periodically she notices that, in the persistent dynamism of her busy life, she is responding automatically to people and events, and as a consequence is missing both the opportunities to let go and have real fun with people, and the occasions when she really needs to devote special attention to some issue.

Finally, there is a substantial group of clients for whom Zero Balancing only gradually becomes their main form of therapy. They go to an acupuncturist, masseur, reflexologist, or chiropractor, who happens also to be qualified in Zero Balancing. The practitioner starts to use a bit of Zero Balancing along with their other work, finds that it helps, and over time does more and more of it at each session. I will look more closely at all these kinds of clients and what benefits they can expect, but first I want to describe a typical session of Zero Balancing.

. . . .

talking

This starts in the normal way with a conversation about the client's medical history. Mainly this is for safety's sake: in some circumstances Zero Balancing may not be appropriate at all. When the client has a recent history of epilepsy, for example, the practitioner simply can't know what might bring on a fit, so it is better not to do a session. Other information might also lead the practitioner to vary her work significantly. The energy body of a client who eats very little or who practises meditation for long periods of time can often be very sensitive, and it is safer to work quickly – holding fulcrums for half the normal time or less.

The conversation will also cover what it is the client wants from the session. In many cases this is straightforward – relief of pain, or relaxation from stress and so on. However sometimes the issue may be more complex. As mentioned before, a person may report that he doesn't feel right, or feels unsupported in his life or is suffering from the break-up of a relationship. Certainly, Zero Balancing can help in all these cases, but the practitioner will want to explore a little before starting to work. Not with the intention of delving into the psychology of the issue, but simply to find a way of summarizing it in such a way that the work will have the most effect. This summary is important because it creates a 'frame' for the work. I put the word frame in inverted commas because it is an image, rather as 'donkey' is an image. The frame of a painting, which appears not to do anything has, in fact, a vital function. It separates what is included in the painting from what isn't. Applying the analogy to a Zero Balancing session, the frame enables the practitioner to decide what to put in the session and what to leave out. After all, there are many kinds of fulcrums which can be done in many places on the body – and all of them can be done a number of times and held for different lengths of time. The frame guides the practitioner in making all these choices. More generally, it suggests a way of working so that all the separate pieces of work she does form one harmonious whole.

. . . .

the protocol

The work is done with the client fully clothed; he just takes off his shoes and his belt, if he is wearing one. This is unusual for bodywork, but it does have advantages. For one thing, many people's donkeys feel a little alarmed and vulnerable when they are in underclothes only. For another, it is actually much easier for the practitioner to move her hands under the body if it is clothed. Unless skin is oiled, the friction between the skin of the two people tends to ruck the soft tissue of the client's back and make it harder to put in a clear fulcrum at just the right place. Lastly, there is no difficulty in feeling energy and structure through clothing; in fact, cutting out the information conveyed by the client's skin tone helps to keep a clearer focus.

The work is then done in a set sequence, which is called the 'protocol' in the language of Zero Balancing. The following description of the work follows the sequence of the protocol. Experienced practitioners will occasionally deviate from the protocol when they sense, for example, that it would be better, for a particular client, to work on the neck before the sacro-iliac joint, reversing the normal sequence – but they have all come to appreciate the value of sticking to the normal order of work in most cases.

It starts with the client sitting on the couch. The practitioner stands behind him, rests her hands briefly on his shoulders and then, with her thumbs, touches each rib briefly, first one side then the other, moving steadily down the back to about the ninth rib. This is a form of evaluation, giving the practitioner an initial sense of energy and structure in the rib cage, but more important is that it gives her an ideal opportunity to make a donkey connection. The first thing a donkey needs is to feel safe, and this is a safe area. So at this first stage of the session there is much more chance of a genuine meeting with the client's donkey here than anywhere else. And it helps too that the natural response to pressure on the back is to counterbalance it by leaning against it. Getting into that habit right from the outset makes it easier for the donkey to do so later with unaccustomed fulcrums. Sometimes, of course, even that natural impulse to lean is overridden; the back stays rigid and tight, or the client sways forward, pushed by even the gentle pressure on his back. Either of these responses alerts the practitioner to the fact that she is going to have to be very patient and precise in her work if she is to make that all-important donkey connection.

Next comes an evaluation which involves a gentle rotation of the arms. I am not going to describe how this is done, instead I am going to explain what it does: 'what', rather than 'how', is always my focus. This evaluation gives the practitioner a good indication of whether or not there are restrictions in two places; in the shoulder joint itself and in the way the scapula floats on the rib cage. This also gives some indication of the state of the costo-vertebral joints of those ribs which lie under the scapula. Finally, in this opening section of the protocol, the practitioner evaluates the movement in the sacro-iliac joint on both sides.

After this the client lies on his back on the couch, head supported by a small pillow if that is more comfortable, arms relaxed and hands resting somewhere on his abdomen. The practitioner picks up the client's feet and puts in a half moon. A fascinating moment, this, and a privileged one. It's like opening a window on who the person really is. This first fulcrum speaks volumes about the unique way that energy and structure are manifest in this individual human being, and something is revealed which may not be known to any other person in the world. To give you a flavour of what I mean, here are just a few examples taken from the endless variety. It may feel as if the curve of the half moon flows smoothly and steadily all the way up the spine, bringing a gentle smile to the face of the client as it arrives at the head. In contrast, it may feel as if the curve stops abruptly at the sacro-iliac joint, almost as if there were a hinge there where two flat planes of the body intersect. As traction is applied, the practitioner may be surprised by the amount of slack, the body seeming to stretch a long way without shifting at all on the couch, or there may be practically no slack at all. The legs may feel much lighter, or much heavier, than seems likely from the client's body weight; one side may feel heavier than the other, or less flexible. Some clients react instantly, with a smile or a grimace or a sigh, others show no sign that anything is happening at all.

Whatever happens, the practitioner's attitude remains the same. There is no judgement. No result is right or wrong, better or worse. No response, or lack of response, is right or wrong. This is absolutely crucial. As soon as any judgement creeps in, it whispers to the practitioner that she knows how the client ought to be, what he needs, and so on. This does more than get in the way; it stops the client getting what he needs, and may, because the practitioner starts to work towards some goal, actually make things worse. Instead of judgement, there is a more interesting attitude. It is a mixture of acceptance and absorption. Again, I can't help thinking of a musical analogy; it's a bit like the attitude of a conductor. He works with what is – the music as written – and it is precisely by remaining as faithful to that as he can that he brings out its own essential quality and relates its complex patterns and relationships. And as he works he is utterly absorbed in it, holding the pulse and rhythm, balancing the different instruments, leading at the same time as he is being led, noticing everything. It is like this for the practitioner. There is a remarkable synthesis between leading, while at the same time being led by the client. It's actually a benign circle; the clarity and accuracy of the practitioner's work creates an environment in which the client can give authentic messages about what work is needed – which in turn enables the practitioner to work more accurately, and so on and so on. So that first half moon sets the circle in motion, and the practitioner starts the process of leading and being led.

Next she evaluates the sacro-iliac joint again and puts in a fulcrum, or fulcrums. The protocol then takes her to the lower back and she evaluates it all, from about the tenth rib, through the lumbar spine, back to the sacro-iliac joint. It is better to evaluate the whole area before starting to put in any fulcrums because the practitioner needs to feel what is really needed. Are there two distinct places of densely held energy? If so, she will probably want to concentrate on them – by which I mean that she will put in a fulcrum on each, re-evaluate and put in another fulcrum if necessary. Or is there tension all down one side? In which case she may choose to put in a series of relatively quick fulcrums over the whole area before re-evaluating. As her fingers move down the lumbar spine, noticing where a fulcrum would be welcome, she marks such places with a slight pause or a slight extra pressure of the fingers. This is really a message to the client's donkey, 'Don't worry, I know you want me to work there and I'll be back.' It is so lovely, this small act of recognition. In all sorts of situations in life – at work, in big family gatherings – it feels so good when somebody notices how we are. Someone sees that we're getting frustrated at being interrupted when we speak, and stops others doing it – thereby offering respect to us and what we have to say. Someone spots that we're getting cold and brings us a pullover, or it may just be a glance of sympathy when something has been said or done which hurts us, or perhaps a smile of encouragement at a difficult time. Simply being affirmed in this way makes us feel better; so it is with marking the spot that is asking for attention in a Zero Balancing session. And, of course, it helps the donkey to feel it is in safe hands.

Now the practitioner comes to the hip joint, immediately below the sacro-iliac joint. Here she repeats the basic format of evaluation, fulcrum, re-evaluation. The fulcrum here is a strong one, working from the longest bone in the body and through a very stable joint, and it will be felt through the sacro-iliac joint and often up through the spine as well. The natural next step is to evaluate and place fulcrums into the feet, grounding all that has been done so far on the lower half of the body. A half moon from the feet afterwards helps to settle everything in its new state and signals to the donkey that no more will be done there for a while.

Work on the upper half of the body is done with the practitioner sitting on a chair close to the client's head. As she sits down she will ask the client how he is. She is not so much interested in the content of the reply, but she is very alert to how he replies. She realizes that politeness demands that the client will usually say 'fine' or words to that effect, but what the client almost certainly cannot control is the tone and timbre of his voice as he replies. These are important indicators of how the energy body is responding to the work. Again, there is no judgement, but it provides another lead for the practitioner. If, for example, the voice is fuller, stronger and richer than before, she can be pretty sure that the energy body has been stimulated and strengthened by the work so far – and she will probably carry on as before. But if the voice is dull and listless, this is a sign that the energy body is losing rather than gaining vitality. The practitioner is probably not touching at interface, or isn't making a donkey connection, or both. The pacing of the session may be too slow for the donkey, which is flagging because the journey seems aimless and endless. In response, the practitioner will make her touch clearer and firmer, really engaging the structure, and working more vigorously to re-charge the energy body.

She then evaluates the whole of the upper back, working with her hands under the body, and all the motions of the neck. This is done in one piece because of the close functional relationship of neck to upper back, and again she will mark places which seem to want a fulcrum. Following the evaluation come the fulcrums, then re-evaluation and, if necessary, more fulcrums on both the upper back and neck.

In deciding how many fulcrums to put in, the practitioner is guided by a number of considerations. Early on in her training these are the rules of thumb which she remembers. As she becomes more practised, they become instinctive knowledge gathered from her fingertips. One consideration is the overall balance of the session itself. Like any other kind of session, a Zero Balancing session has a beginning, a middle and an end; but the middle rarely comes half way through the allotted time. What is meant by the middle is the area of work on that part of the body where the most powerful change can take place. I will explain later how the practitioner recognizes this, but for now the point is that it may be found at any time – in the first few minutes or near the end. If it has come near the beginning of the session, then the practitioner will tend to work on the upper back in such a way as to help it to integrate and adapt to that important change elsewhere. That is, she may do quite a lot of fulcrums, to cover the area, but will not hold any of them for more than a few seconds; if she repeats them at all, she will tend to do so only once. However, if she hasn't got to the middle by now, and she feels some places in this area which seem to have a lot of held energy, then she might well choose to put in only one or two fulcrums, at least on her first pass, and hold them longer than usual. It may be that work on one of these will turn out to be the key fulcrum of the session. The protocol gives an extremely helpful order of work, but it says nothing about the kind of work to be done at any one place. It certainly shouldn't be taken as implying that every area should receive the same number or kind of fulcrums.

The frame provides a criterion of how to work too. With experience, a practitioner's fingers can tell whether the energy held in a particular place has been there for a long time or not. If the practitioner finds a spot on the upper back which seems to her to hold the energy of some very old trauma, then whether or not she chooses to work there might well depend on the frame. If the frame was to ease a pain in the lower back, caused by some recent accident, she will probably pass it by. If, on the other hand, the frame was to release the unexpressed grief at the loss of a loved one in childhood, then she will pay it close attention, perhaps putting in two or more fulcrums which she holds a little longer than usual.

Over and above these considerations is the donkey connection itself, and the practitioner's attitude of acceptance and absorption. These are a practitioner's most sure guides, and they lead her to an instinctive, but trained, response to the client's needs.

The work on this part of the body is completed with a half moon from the head, which serves to integrate all the work previously done. The session closes with three further integrating half moons. One on the rib cage, done towards the feet, and another on the pelvis, in the same direction, will both serve to align the spine as a whole. The last half moon is from the feet, and will feel very different from the first, opening one of the session. This time, it will co-ordinate all the work that has been done and convey a sense of closure and completion. Sometimes, in addition, the practitioner will hold the feet in her hands for a few moments, with wrists crossed. This helps to re-establish the internal energy flow engendered by walking and prepare the client's energy body for moving again. She sees the client safely off the couch, and may suggest that he stands still for a few moments to get used to being upright again. He then walks up and down the room a few times to get used to the new feeling of his body. The whole session will have taken somewhere between 20 and 40 minutes.

. . . .

the client's experience

Zero Balancing certainly feels different. Whatever other form of bodywork the client may have had, this is a new experience. His mind will register some of the things that make it so, but for most new clients the most remarkable thing is that nothing much seems to have happened. They will often start to get off the couch, saying politely that it was very nice, and you can hear the unexpressed end of the sentence, '...but I don't think it's done anything.' Then, as they stand, a puzzled look comes over their face. 'That's odd,' it seems to say, 'I do actually feel a bit...hard to say really.' The puzzled look is replaced by a kind of concentration, as the mind scans the interior trying to find out what's gone on.

One reason why they think nothing much has happened is that the work is so gentle. There is none of the sudden shock of manipulation, as with osteopathy or chiropractic. There is none of the repeated strong pressure of massage, or stronger pressure of Rolfing. And it doesn't hurt. Occasionally, the practitioner may put in a fulcrum on a place which feels sore to the touch. In a way, this hurts, but it is by no means an unpleasant feeling; in fact the client often feels that this spot has been crying out for help and it is a relief that it is being attended to. There is an American phrase for this; they say 'it hurts good' (as opposed to 'it hurts bad'). As I explain later in this chapter, those moments when a fulcrum 'hurts good' can be occasions for profound healing.

In addition, compared to most other forms of bodywork, the amount of time the body is actually being worked on is very small. Fulcrums are in place for only somewhere between five and ten minutes in a whole session. This figure is perhaps a bit misleading, because the evaluations and re-evaluations also have an effect on structure and energy, although a lot less than fulcrums. Even including them, the practitioner's hands are probably only on the client for about half the time of the session. So the client's experience that he has not been worked on much is accurate.

This is another of the wonderful paradoxes of Zero Balancing. The pauses, when no work is being done, are at least as important as the fulcrums. In fact, stillness is at the heart of this therapy. Remember how in the stillness of the fulcrum the client can move to a new configuration of energy and structure. The stillness between fulcrums is another aspect of the same idea. It mirrors a basic dynamic of the body. Between the in-breath and the out-breath is a pause; between the contractions of a heartbeat is a pause; between each day is the pause of sleep. A sequence of action and stillness is a fundamental rhythm, and work which respects this is more easily assimilated. Think of a fulcrum as like a meal; the body has to digest it before it can cope with another one. After a big nourishing meal, the last thing you want is to be rushed off to another one. Putting in a series of powerful fulcrums without pausing between them is a bit like piling in rich meals, one on top of the other.

One of the practitioner's skills is to recognize how long to pause; to sense very accurately how long it takes for each fulcrum to be digested. There is a lot of variety between clients, and there can be a big difference between fulcrums in the same session. In some cases the practitioner may feel it is best to do a whole sequence of short fulcrums, for example right up the upper back, before pausing at the end. In other cases she will leave a few seconds between each fulcrum; that will be enough. But when she realizes that a particular fulcrum has formed the middle of the session, and the whole of the client's energy and structure are re-organizing profoundly, the pause may last a few minutes. These pauses are very highly charged times, and it would not only be a waste of a wonderful opportunity to interrupt them prematurely, it could also be quite distressing to the client. He may not know what is going on, but he knows he is in a state which is precious and not to be disturbed. It is a kind of reverie, almost a dreamlike state. Time stands still; it might be more accurate to say that in this state time doesn't exist.

So the overall experience is of very gentle work punctuated by some moments which hurt good and many pauses. There will also be occasional lapses into some deep state – more about this later in the chapter.

. . . .

after the session

The initial responses from clients are very varied. Here are some quotations from my own practice.

> 'It seemed as if there was a concrete square in my back, and it's now all light.'

> 'Well…for the first time for weeks I'm without that constant dull pain in my left leg.'

> 'It's such a relief to release the grief… I knew it was there but…'

> 'I had no idea how tense I was.'

> 'My top half used to feel heavy and my bottom half light – now it's the other way round, which feels much better.'

These are all positive reactions and there are exceptions, of course. I have had one client who may have felt worse after the session; at any rate he rushed away and never came back. And another who I know felt worse – I describe his case later. There are some clients who appear not to feel any change at all, and indeed, nothing much may have happened. I will discuss this later too. Very often, the client doesn't feel the change, or perhaps doesn't trust the reality of the feeling of change, until a few minutes after the end of the session, when he has walked up and down for a bit. Then, gradually, it starts to dawn on him. What is happening, I think, is a kind of slow translation process. It takes time for the mind to receive the new sensations from the body, time to interpret them into a conceptual category, and time to formulate those into words. For many people, only when that has happened will they allow themselves to believe what they are feeling. However, some people register immediately exactly what has happened. I always remember one of my very first clients, an artist who had been unable to paint for nearly a year; a block which had caused her immense distress. She opened her eyes as she sat up on the couch and said, with wonder in her voice, 'I can see again'. Later she told me in that moment she knew that was the block: because she had been depressed, but hadn't quite realized it, the world had become grey, cloudy and foggy, and there was really nothing to paint. I have one of her paintings now, in my treatment room, and it is the first thing that clients see as they sit up after a session.

Even when a session has brought about big changes, its initial effects may not be felt for a day or so. It seems to take the body time to settle into its new patterns and orientation. While it is doing so the client may even feel a dip in his energy levels, or a slight aggravation of pain in certain places, which may last for a few hours. Whether or not this occurs, the client usually starts to feel much better within 24 hours. In some ways, he has to be cautious of this. A man in his mid-seventies, very active and full of life, came to me for a session because for the past six months he had been in so much pain from his lower back that he had been unable to walk more than a few hundred yards. I saw him again after a week and asked him how he was. 'No better', he replied. Fortunately I was, by then, sufficiently experienced to ask a few more questions, and it turned out that two days after the session he had felt so good that he had gone for a two mile walk. In other words, it is as well not to expose a new state of being to such a severe test. You wouldn't plant a young tree and leave it exposed to the winds without a supporting stake, or take a person who has just given up smoking to a stressful party full of smokers.

With long-term or chronic issues, it may take a long while for the full effects of the change to be seen. The healing process may be at work, but it takes time. Often, in these kinds of cases, the practitioner will suggest that a few sessions might be appropriate; each building on and reinforcing the work of the one before. I once worked with a psychotherapist who had had a migraine every few weeks for over 20 years and who was naturally doubtful that any form of bodywork could relieve their frequency or intensity. I suggested to her that we made a commitment to three sessions, each a fortnight apart. In part, my thinking was that it was a long-standing condition so it would be sensible to have a few sessions and to give each one time to settle before adding another. And partly that it would take her donkey at least one session to relax and trust that this work might be helpful. She wasn't sure that there was any change after the first session. In the week after the second, she felt the familiar signs of a migraine coming on, but it didn't develop, and since the third session, over 18 months ago now, she hasn't had a migraine at all.

There is another kind of outcome to a session. It is that the client feels really well. Even as I write this I can hear it falling a little flat, and it seems to me such a shame that it should do so. In our culture, we focus so much on illness or disease that we undervalue being genuinely well. We think the task of therapy of all kinds is the removal of what we don't want, rather than the fostering and enhancement of what we do. But the ability to live life to the full, to have the capacity to respond vigorously to a joyful occasion – or even to a sad and painful one – is a great gift. With that ability goes the confidence and clarity to make good choices in life; those which will lead a person to make the best use of their talents and realize their dreams. Creativity flourishes, fear loses some of its grip and the burdens of the past can be put down more easily. With all this comes benefits for others too. Someone in this kind of state is a joy to be with and, when called upon to help, is more present for the person in need. More and more clients are allowing themselves to come for Zero Balancing because it makes them feel really well.

Some clients seem to get no benefit at all, and I could leave this issue by simply saying that not everything works all the time on everyone – which is true – but I think it is more interesting to look at some of the different reasons for this.

One possibility is that the practitioner didn't make a donkey connection. This manifests itself in all sorts of ways; missing the places which really needed a fulcrum, doing too much, or too little work, getting the pacing of the session wrong and so on. It isn't always easy, and there are plenty of ways to go wrong. The better the practitioner, the wider the range of people she can treat successfully, but we all have our limits. Another possibility is that this kind of work is clearly inappropriate for the client's problem. It would be unrealistic to think it could help with an enlarged prostate gland, bowel problems or psoriasis. Having said that, there are some surprises. I had no idea that it would help with premature hair loss, but it has. I now suppose, though I didn't guess at the time, that the condition was caused mainly by stress. This is a complex issue, and I shall cover it in the next section of this chapter.

There can be times when, during a session, the practitioner is sure that there is a significant change taking place. And this is confirmed when the client comes off the couch. He looks taller, clearer. His face is a better colour and there is a sparkle in his eyes. He looks at you with a soft smile. The atmosphere in the room is quiet and concentrated. You feel good about the session. Taken all together, these signs tell a story which it is hard to doubt. Yet the next time you see him, he looks the same as before, and reports no improvement in his condition. On one such occasion the client reported angrily that he felt he had been 'messed up' (this is the example I referred to earlier). I was astonished; so sure had I been that it had gone very well, indeed much better than usual. What happened, I think, was that the client had indeed had a brief experience of feeling very much better, and that experience was threatening. So he dismissed, discounted or rejected it. Generalizing, I think it is fair to say that even though the client may want to be well, unconsciously the change it would entail is too big. For some people, being unwell is so much a part of their lives that they cannot imagine it otherwise. Being well might involve changes at work – if his job is organized around a disability – or in his relationship, if his wife's reaction to his problems is to look after him a lot. It might involve changes in his self-image if he thinks of himself as a person who is ill. Sometimes people in these kinds of situations come for a session simply because they need to believe they have done everything possible to be healed.

Finally, in any discussion of the effects of any therapy, it is essential to acknowledge that the work forms only a very tiny part of the client's life, and the circumstances of that life may have vastly more influence on what happens than anything the practitioner might do. It is unrealistic, and arrogant, to believe otherwise.

. . . .

healing

In the previous section I described the kinds of changes that happen quite routinely after a session; they are the kinds of outcomes you would expect. An alleviation of pain, an improvement in walking, a feeling of well-being.

But Zero Balancing can work at an entirely different level too. It has the potential to heal old wounds, whether physical, emotional, mental or spiritual. This is a big claim, but it is not an idle one. There is one feature of Zero Balancing, one thing that can happen in a session, which makes this a genuine possibility.

I mentioned earlier that a client may sometimes lapse into a reverie, a deep dreamlike state. It is in this state that such healing can take place. I will first explain what it is and then how it is brought about.

William James, the great American philosopher and psychologist, wrote in 1901, 'Our normal waking consciousness...is but one special type of consciousness, whilst all about it, parted from it by the filmiest of screens, there lie potential forms of consciousness entirely different. We may go through life without suspecting their existence; but apply the requisite stimulus, and at a touch there they are in all their completeness...' (William James, *Varieties of Religious Experience*, p. 374).

There is nothing strange or esoteric about these other states of consciousness; most of us have experienced them. As a small child, awake in bed at night, I could see my room as infinitely large, stretching endlessly into the distance, or as minutely small – the whole of it, with me included, fitting in a thimble. William Blake, the artist and poet, to take a rather more grand example, 'Sauntering along...looks up and sees a tree filled with angels, bright angelic wings bespangling every bough like stars' (Peter Ackroyd, *Blake*, p. 23). Einstein reported that he just saw how space was, and wrote down his world-changing equation as simply a description of what he'd seen. And the *Revelation of St John the Divine*, in the New Testament, is a breathtaking description of a very extended other state of consciousness. Few people have not had some such experience, although many will have ignored or forgotten it.

In such a state, the normal thinking mind is somehow absent. If it were present and functioning it would preserve the 'filmiest of screens' and we would never even realize that we could, indeed, see the world differently. Sometimes, we do get a glimpse; then, with extraordinary speed, the mind filters, interprets and judges the impressions we are receiving and tells us that 'this isn't really happening' or 'it's some trick of the light, some hallucination'. It does this in the interests of keeping us normal in the daily world. All the accounts written by those who have experienced another state — and there are huge numbers of them — point to the fact that in such a state a person can see, hear, feel, and know what is beyond the mind's comprehension, and beyond its capacity to plan and organize our actions. A common report, for example, is that there is no difference between one human being and another, nor between humans, animals, rocks or even stars. It is all one. What is impossible, unimaginable even, in normal consciousness is perfectly possible in one of these other states.

And that is where healing comes in. In his normal state a client has this pain or that sense of failure; this buried childhood grief or that desperate depression. But in another state he may not have it. In other words, being in a state where he doesn't have it, and experiencing being without it, acts as a fulcrum. His body, mind and spirit can re-organize around that experience of being without it. So when he returns to normal waking consciousness, it is no longer there: he is healed.

Certainly, this is a theory. But it is a theory which accounts for the fact that profound healing of this kind does take place — every doctor, let alone complementary therapist, knows of examples — and that it is often associated with the client falling into a deep dreamlike state in which time seems to stand still.

There are many ways to access such a state. Hallucinogenic drugs are used for this purpose. For thousands of years people have done it through meditation. Prisoners deprived of sleep or of light experience it. These are all examples of what William James meant by 'the requisite stimulus'; that intervention which 'parts the screens'. And, judging from the considerable numbers of reports from clients of Zero Balancing, a fulcrum can be a requisite stimulus.

There are two reasons to believe that fulcrums can have this effect. All these stimuli – drugs, sensory deprivation and meditation – do the same thing; they bypass the normal thinking mind. And a fulcrum can do exactly the same thing, in a number of ways. One is by holding a foundation or semi-foundation joint into a configuration it has never been in before. The mind just won't know what to make of that. It can tell, from the energetic and structural shifts taking place, in response to the fulcrum, that something is going on. But deprived of reports from the area of the fulcrum itself, for there are no nerves or musculature there, it doesn't know what is going on. The mind has no way of finding out, or, because it is all new, no way of working it out. So it gives up. And that opens the door, parts the screens, accesses other states. That is why the client experiences this as a reverie, a dreamlike state in which time stands still; for a few moments the mind is not relaying its constant messages of 'do this, avoid that, think about this, notice that'. So there is no sequence either; no first thought and then second thought, no 'do this and then that'. It is exactly what has been taught by meditators for thousands of years; it is when the mind gives up that we see other realms of being, other realities.

Another way in which a fulcrum can cause the mind to give up for a few moments is to give it contradictory messages. If it can't work out what to make of an input, is really baffled as to how to categorize it, and the input is insistent and cannot be ignored, then it might just stop working until it has something normal to grasp onto again. A touch which hurts good can do this. On the one hand, it hurts – category, 'avoid this or complain'; on the other hand, we have been craving touch in that place for ages and it feels good – category 'accept this, take as much of it as you can'. The inconsistency between these two is so total, that no resolution or accommodation is possible. So the mind shuts down until it's over.

Interestingly, there are parallels in ordinary life. If you have a deeply held belief – for example that a loved one is a good and honest man, and then you receive information which flatly contradicts that belief, what do you do? Well, you might refuse to believe the information, cast doubt on it, re-examine the evidence for your belief that he is a good man and so on – all ways of trying to wriggle out of the difficulty – and one of these ways might work for you. But sometimes the difficulty really persists; you cannot stop believing he is a good man and the information is true. What can happen to people in this situation is that they think they are going mad. They say that they are losing their mind and, in a way, they are right; the mind cannot deal with the contradiction so it packs up, briefly. Those who have been suddenly and unexpectedly bereaved can have a similar reaction; they can't believe it, but it's true. And quite often at all these times of overwhelming stress to the mind, the screen parts and people have profound experiences which are not possible in 'normal life'. Some of these can be healing too; an awareness that a deceased loved one is 'safe and well' or 'with the angels' may be absolutely real to the bereaved and deeply consoling too.

To put all this in context, these altered states of consciousness are common, but not routine, in Zero Balancing sessions. When it happens it is unmistakable, for both client and practitioner. A wonderful atmosphere permeates the room and there is a different quality to the relationship between the two people; it is as if they are sharing something. What happens in those moments cannot be predicted. It may be some healing, it may be an insight into a difficulty in the client's life, it may be an experience of the divine. All these have been reported on many occasions. Nor can it even be adequately described afterwards; the mind was not there to record it and words exist only in the everyday state of consciousness. It is a mystery and a gift.

the art

· ·

*When we have no thought of achievement, no thought of self,
we are true beginner... This is also the real secret of the arts:
always be a beginner.* (Shunryu Suzuki, *Zen Mind, Beginner's
Mind*, pp. 21–22)

In this chapter, I focus on the art of Zero Balancing and the way it develops
in the practitioner, rather than on the nature of the work and its effect on
a client. How does her skill as a practitioner turn into an art? How does
that art enable her to work with a client's pain, depression or feelings
of worthlessness? And what effect does the practice of this art have on
her? These are the issues of this chapter, and although I treat them in
the context of Zero Balancing, much of what I cover will be relevant to
practitioners of other therapies.

As the practitioner's skills develop, something else develops too. Instead
of the skills being merely actions which are performed as taught,
following the instructor's directions and copying his movements,
they become internalized; that is, they become instinctive and almost
automatic responses to the development of the session as a whole, and
to the changing relationship of energy and structure in the client. Rather
than evaluating and putting in fulcrums as taught, and just hoping that
they are having the desired effect, the practitioner begins to know what
is happening and how best to adjust what she is doing and how she
is doing it to enhance and refine her work. She begins to develop her
own style of working. Again, a musical metaphor comes to mind. While
a pianist is learning the skills needed to play a sonata, there is little
scope for her interpretation of the piece, but once she has mastered
those skills, she will play it in her own way. If you hear it played first by
someone else, and then by her, it will be recognizably the same piece of
music but it will sound significantly different. It is very much the same
with Zero Balancing. Two experienced practitioners can do a half moon

from the feet and they will both clearly be half moons, and they will both balance energy and structure, but they will feel very different. It is almost as if each has a person's signature on it. And each person's touch is highly individual too. Again, it will clearly be a touch at interface, and it will make a donkey connection, but it will still be unique.

. . . .

feeling energy

It is exciting and awe-inspiring, the moment when you actually feel a movement of energy in another human being. Up to that moment, the mind has all kinds of explanations: 'It doesn't actually exist – these people are kidding themselves'. Or an inner voice says, 'Well of course you can't do it; you're not sensitive' or, 'Sure you felt something, but you were imagining things, making it up in order to be part of the group'. But in the moment it is first felt, all this is swept away as simply irrelevant. In my mind's eye I can see even now a highly respected 50-year-old company director jumping up and down, waving her arms like an ostrich trying to fly, shouting, 'I felt it, it's there', over and over again. That's the excitement. It is awe-inspiring because it is a glimpse into an aspect of how the world works – it must have been similar for the first people to look at a snowflake or a worm under a microscope. Suddenly they could see what it was really like; the orderliness of it all.

To get to a point where you are able to feel energy, you have to practise. Not because it is difficult or because there is a particular or right way of doing it, but mainly to learn to trust what it is you are feeling. It is a matter of educating the mind to allow you to register the sensations as valid. 'But surely', the mind says, 'what you are feeling is so subjective – how can you possibly do work on that basis, let alone work on another human being?'

This is the mind struggling to re-assert control of the situation. It isn't true. The feeling is not subjective; no more than a radio picking up sound waves is subjective. You are simply picking up energy waves in your hands, and they will feel more or less the same to anyone else who has learned to trust the feelings in her hands. I say 'more or less' because those with more experience get more information, and clearer information too. If you can find some way of conveying what these energy waves feel like, other practitioners will recognize your description, again, more or less. There may well be interesting discussion around exactly what it feels like, but even so, contradictory views are extremely rare.

Once you are prepared to trust your feelings, and you start to get more specific information through your hands, you start to notice what happens when you put in a fulcrum. Figure 13 gives some visual analogues for what a half moon from the feet can feel like. All of these, except perhaps the last one – where the energy just keeps on flowing out of the top of the client's head – are pretty common. At first, you might use this feeling of energy simply as a benchmark. Does the client's energy feel better – clearer, more coherent – at the end of the session than at the start? That is a useful measure of the effectiveness of a session. Then, you might start to use the information to influence how you work. To take the example of Figure 13 (d), my instinct would be to make the fulcrum extremely clear, forceful and deliberate as the existing force field is jumbled and somewhat chaotic. I want to emphasize, and this holds true for what follows in this chapter, that using a clear and forceful fulcrum is not a decision I would make by thinking it out. It would be my trained, instinctual reaction to the sensation I feel in my own hands. No doubt my mind plays some part in all this, but as best I can I leave it to be quiet, and rely on the practised response of my hands. Occasionally, of course, the mind will butt in and whisper, 'Why don't you try it with more curve?' or, 'You need to use less traction.' If that happens I can't altogether ignore it, but I don't decide, consciously, to accept or reject the advice; I convey it to my hands and let them choose what to do.

In the case of a simple lifting fulcrum, Figure 14 shows some representations of what you might feel (the arrow is the fulcrum; the parallel lines are the bone). These are all fairly common too. Often, while a fulcrum is in place, you start to feel movement under your finger, which is represented in Figure 14 (e).

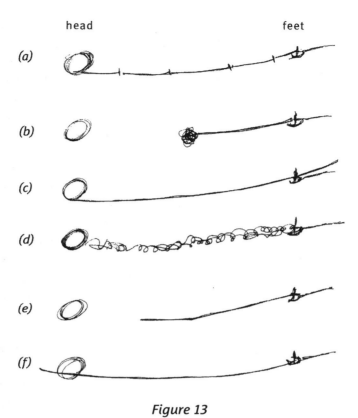

head   feet

(a)

(b)

(c)

(d)

(e)

(f)

Figure 13

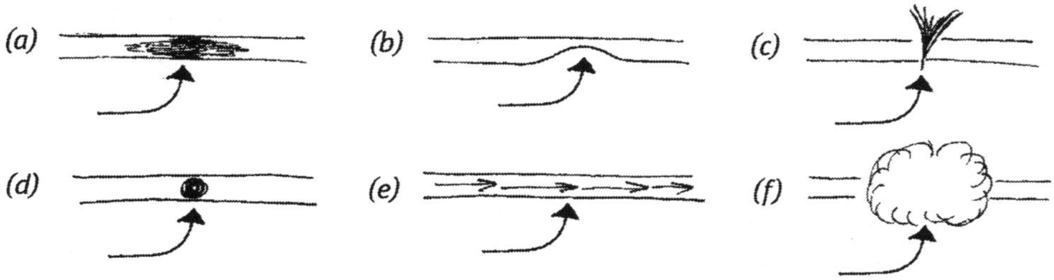

(a)   *(b)*   *(c)*

(d)   *(e)*   *(f)*

Figure 14

Being able to feel energy through a fulcrum opens up another level of practice. Any fulcrum will have an effect where it is placed; but it can also have an effect elsewhere too. It is quite easy to feel, for example, that the main effect of work on held energy in the middle of the back will be on restrictions in movement in the client's neck; the feeling is prompted, at any rate for the novice, by the knowledge that the trapezius muscle connects the two. And that opens the possibility of putting in a fulcrum in one place deliberately to affect another, rather as a kite flyer moves the kite by pulling at the end of the string. In principle, given that all parts of the body are structurally and energetically interconnected, this makes perfect sense. In practice, the issue is finding the specific place from which change can occur at the other end of the string. In engineering terms, it is finding the place of maximum leverage. In energetic terms it is a bit like finding the boulder that is causing a whirlpool downstream; or, to use another image, knowing exactly what to say and exactly when to say it in order to change the atmosphere at an unproductive and sterile meeting.

It isn't altogether easy to say how a practitioner feels that a restriction in one place can be eased by a fulcrum in another; perhaps this is at the borderline between skill and art. At any rate, it isn't something which is worked out rationally, although the explanation may come later. I once worked on a man who had had a strong and persistent headache for some time. As soon as I started to put a fulcrum into his left foot, I knew I had the headache under my hand; only later did I realize that the onset of the headaches coincided with an injury to his foot a few years earlier. The best I can do is to point to two indicators. First, when evaluating or putting in the fulcrum, there is a strong sensation that this is a highly charged area; a lot of energy is collected, or even imprisoned there. You get something like this feeling when you walk into a room where two people have just had a row – or just fallen in love. Secondly, as you start to put in the fulcrum, you can feel that there is a response in some other part of the body; it really is like the tug of a kite at the end of line as it is caught by a puff of wind. Sometimes, you can see a confirmation of your sensation; that part of the body twitches or stirs, the client may scratch or rub it; all unconscious responses to a change occurring in that place. Going back to my client with a headache, I suppose that what I actually felt was that the energy in his foot was highly charged, and that I was starting to connect with some tension, restriction, or issue which was a long way away – I don't honestly know how precise I could be about exactly where I was feeling it, because, knowing all about his headache, I suppose that I immediately put two and two together and made four.

These are all examples of feeling energy conveyed by one fulcrum. Another stage of learning is when the practitioner starts to feel the overall state of a client's energy. This can be picked up at specific times – in an evaluation, during a fulcrum, or even when the practitioner is getting her hands in place to work – but for me, it is more often a kind of dawning realization. I have felt something doing an early evaluation, and only when I have felt it again, perhaps a few times, do I realize that it is an overall pattern, a general energy state. There may be a great deal of vibration in the body, somewhat like a sustained high note of a violin, or, by contrast, its energy may be rather slow and dulled in quality. Quite often it may feel as if there are two energy zones in the body; one full and the other empty. Occasionally there may be a place which just seems empty, as if it is uninhabited. It seems that when people have had a traumatic experience which particularly affects some part of the body, they may take their awareness, and hence their energy, away from that place in order to protect themselves from experiencing the pain there.

Dr Oliver Sacks, the well-known author and Professor of Clinical Neurology, describes his own experience of this phenomenon in a book called *A Leg to Stand On*. Although his badly broken leg had healed perfectly, energetically all was not well. He woke one morning to find another person's leg in his bed. Dozy from sleep, but outraged by this intrusion, he threw the leg out – only to find himself on the floor. He still did not associate cause and effect – so he did it again, with exactly the same result. What is especially interesting is that even when he had worked out what was happening, and that it was indeed his own leg, he was still unable to feel it as his own; the disassociation could not be restored by his rational conscious mind. All this has been put, more succinctly and more poetically, by Emmanuel.

106

Illness exists first
in the non-physical realm
of spiritual need,
emotional confusion,
or mental aberration.
It is never primarily physical.
The body is the reactor.
It vibrates to stress
and is the outward manifestation
of inner turmoil.

(Pat Rodegast and Judith Stanton (eds.), *Emmanuel's Book*, p. 159)

This quotation speaks about how the client's problem or issue may be represented in his body. In a session given by Fritz Smith, for example, the client spoke at the beginning of not being able to walk out into the world with confidence. In his early forties and well over six feet tall, he walked with a stoop and spoke in a thin weak voice. He had always been somewhat shy and retiring, he explained, but he now wanted to be different and to be able to seize the public opportunities which were presenting themselves to him. With no preconceived idea of how this might be mirrored in the client's body, nor where he might find it, Fritz Smith started to work. When he picked up the client's right leg, in order to evaluate the hip joint, there it was in his hands. A clear but very thin and rather fragile line of energy ran down the leg; not strong enough to support this big man's wish to stride out in the world. With a well-placed fulcrum, Fritz could feel energy start to fill the leg, like the tide creeping into an estuary, finding its way to fill the available space.

The same thing can be experienced from the other direction; the practitioner may find a highly specific energetic pattern which strongly suggests a problem or issue in the client's life. Once when Fritz Smith worked on me he found a considerable blockage of energy between the skull and the atlas, the top cervical vertebra. The effect of this was that I was quite unable to glide my head backwards and forwards – the kind of motion that pigeons make when they walk. The rigidity with which I held my head in the forward position made him think of a young man at a military academy. He asked me, 'Did you go to a military school? Did you learn to stand to attention as a young man?' Without pause for thought, I replied, 'I didn't have to go to a military school to learn that; I had to do it at home.' This is not to say that the practitioner needs to know the cause or source of an energy blockage to put in a fulcrum; simply that being able to feel a client's issue as an imbalance of energy and structure, under your hands, enables the practitioner to work very precisely and very powerfully at deep levels; levels which, it is often assumed, are only accessible through extended psychoanalysis.

. . . .

the dance

Fundamentally, the practitioner's attention is in her fingertips. As I described in Chapter 2, this is a key way of achieving and maintaining interface in her touch. However, once she knows how to do this, she can split her attention. To repeat the example I used earlier, it is a little like driving while listening to the radio; attention in the fingertips, like the driver's attention on the road ahead, carries on without deliberate awareness. While her background attention is on the work in her hands, her foreground attention is gathering information which will help her to make that work a more precise and sophisticated response to the client's needs.

One vital use of this split attention is to notice the client's involuntary reactions to the work. Through long experience, Fritz Smith realized that there are some reactions which indicate that a change is taking place, or has just taken place, in the client's energy state. At the simplest level, these show the practitioner that something is happening; that there is a re-organization around a fulcrum. That is helpful because it confirms that she is working at interface and has a donkey connection. At a more subtle level, the reactions speak volumes as to what the client's donkey really needs, and lead the practitioner to respond to those needs with accuracy and delicacy.

One classic response (there are many others) is where the client's breathing becomes very light and shallow – he may even stop breathing for some 10 to 20 seconds – after which he takes a deep in-breath and a big sighing out-breath. What is going on here, what information does it convey, and how does the practitioner make use of that information?

There are two aspects to what is going on. One is that the energetic change is so interesting and important that the client's full attention is focused on it. This is a relatively common experience. Imagine you are gluing together three pieces of a broken china bowl – a bowl which is made of particularly delicate china and which is of great sentimental value. The intensity of the work and the tension of the moment removes your awareness of all outside stimuli which might interfere with it – you don't hear noises in the street, you don't notice that you're getting cold – and very often, you don't breathe either. Similarly, people hold their breath when the moment comes for some important announcement; all the focus is on the one thing – 'Did I win the Oscar?', for example. As soon as the moment is over and the glue holds, or the announcement is made, the body can then breathe again, and the breath will be bigger than usual to make up for the missed breaths. Sometimes, the energetic change continues for a long time; so after a while, however interesting and important it is, the body insists on more oxygen and less carbon dioxide, and a large in-breath is followed by an equally large out-breath.

All of this breathing pattern is entirely involuntary, and that is why it is so valuable for the practitioner. At some point in a session, it may be helpful to ask a client a question, for example asking if the touch is too firm. But the answer could be influenced by the client wishing to say the right thing, being polite or indeed feeling resistant for some reason. But this breath cycle is not under his control. It is, if you like, a response from the client's donkey rather than his mind. So it is a completely reliable guide; donkeys cannot lie, and have absolutely no social skills. The practitioner will know that after a big in-breath followed by a big out-breath, she can release the fulcrum. The work has been done. In fact, to hold onto it after the work has been done doesn't feel good to the client. At best it is irritating, and at worst it feels pressurizing; like being insistently reminded to do something which you've already done. This example, on how long to hold a fulcrum, is just one of the many ways in which the client and practitioner dance together, collaborate – consciously on her part, unconsciously on his – in the work.

A novice Zero Balancing practitioner has to make many decisions in the course of a session, but once she has become really familiar with the protocol, there seem to be very few decisions necessary. This is the phenomenon reported by musicians, writers, dancers, rock climbers and many other kinds of people who become highly skilled at what they do. 'I didn't write the book', said Arthur Ransome, in response to a question about the creation of his best-loved novel, 'It wrote me.' Given a real understanding of the form with which one is working, and an instinctive response to the signs of energetic change – developed by hours of practice – then once the process has started it seems that there is only one way in which it can unfold. The myriad of involuntary signs and signals tell the practitioner what is going on in the session, and she responds to them. The more skilled the practitioner the more she notices, and the more she knows exactly what they mean. And the more effortlessly she dances the dance of that particular client's journey through the protocol and through this opportunity for healing.

. . . .

wellness

When I was just starting to learn Zero Balancing I once saw Fritz Smith briefly before he started a full day's work. He looked well; remarkably well, I thought, for a man in his mid-sixties. I knew I was going to see him again at the end of his day, by which time he would have given ten or more Zero Balancing sessions, and I expected to see a rather different picture. To give full attention to ten separate individuals, quite apart from the sheer physical work involved, would leave him tired, even drained, I supposed. It would have been a long day's work even for a much younger man. But when he came in to the room I was astonished to see that he looked better than before. It looked as if, rather than giving sessions, he had been receiving them. This made a huge impression on me. Although 20 years younger, I was often very weary at the end of a day with patients in my acupuncture practice, and I was surrounded by colleagues who, fairly regularly, felt burned out. I recognized that whatever else he did to be so well, a good deal of his vitality came from doing this work. At the same time as the astonishment came a recognition that this was exactly how it should be; it would have been unbalanced if the work was very beneficial for one person but debilitating to the other. The work had to be consistent with, faithful to, its own principles. What I couldn't see, then, was how this was done; how the practitioner, in the very act of giving a session, could receive as well.

Throughout the previous chapters there have been plenty of indications of how this might work – the mutuality of the donkey connection, for example, implies that the practitioner will share the experience of support which the client receives. But in this chapter I want to give the whole topic the specific attention it deserves. The skills in which a Zero Balancing practitioner is trained, and which lead to this benign outcome, are interesting and important in their own right. But, perhaps more importantly, the essence of them is not confined to Zero Balancing. I think it will be genuinely helpful to all kinds of health care practitioners to reflect on what it is that Zero Balancers do which enables them to feel better at the end of a day's work, and the ways in which the principles can be applied to their own work. This is not to claim that all these skills and principles are unique to Zero Balancing, or that Fritz Smith discovered them. They are probably common to all the masters; those who, whatever kind of therapy they practise, appear to do effortless magic.

One of the features of working with touch is that any strain in the practitioner's body is communicated to the client. Noticing that the client is not comfortable gives the practitioner a strong hint that she should check her own posture. Much of the time, of course, we are unaware of the way we hold our bodies and, out of habit or indifference, we hold them in ways which distort our structure and drain our energy. As I wrote these words, I checked my own posture. My shoulders were hunched, my back was slumped and my legs were crossed, with the foot of the supporting leg lifted and twisted so the heel was off the ground and there was enormous pressure on the ball of the foot. Bizarre!

About half of the work in a Zero Balancing session is done with the practitioner standing. To do this work well, it is essential that she is well-grounded with her weight low in her body. It feels very peculiar to be touched by someone who isn't grounded – almost as if they are a helium-filled balloon and you, the client, are holding them down. You don't quite know if you can manage it, and it feels as if you might drift off with them too. Unnerving. There are all sorts of ways for the practitioner to get grounded. For a start, it helps to have the knees gently flexed; it sinks the body weight down and makes the whole frame more stable. It helps to breathe from the belly rather than the upper chest, and to let the shoulders fall.

The other half of the work is done sitting. Anyone who has watched how many teenagers manage to sit on chairs tilted back on only two legs will know that groundedness is an issue here too. Sitting back in the chair, with the upper body leaning against the chair's back, body weight is dispersed into its seat and out through all four legs in a rather diffuse way. By contrast, if the practitioner sits forward on the chair, so her trunk is directly over its two front legs and her legs are spread to either side, feet planted on the ground taking the weight of the lower legs, the position is very stable and clear and the whole body feels more alert and energized. All these qualities will be reflected in her touch. And if the practitioner spends all day in a posture which is grounded, clear, alert and energized, it isn't so surprising that she feels better at the end of the day.

Another aspect of the same point is avoiding strain or fatigue. It is obvious that a person will feel tired if he spends all day at a desk which is the wrong height, or making awkward stretching movements, or with muscles permanently clenched with the effort of rushing through tasks, and he consistently ignores the complaints of his body. By contrast, a principle of Zero Balancing is that whenever a practitioner feels any strain or fatigue in her hands when evaluating or putting in a fulcrum, she should immediately disconnect. This is actually quite a difficult principle to honour. I well know the feeling of having found a rather elusive place of held energy, putting in a fulcrum which feels just right, and then noticing that my hand is tired or there is tension in my wrist. It is very tempting to say to oneself, 'Well, it's only for a few moments, and I can stand it and the client really needs this fulcrum and anyway I'm not sure I could find this spot again.' But, of course, a fulcrum placed by a tired hand or one which is hurting won't feel good to the client. He may not have any idea why it doesn't feel good, but the touch will lack purpose and clarity – not surprisingly, as much of the practitioner's attention will be on how long she can hold it before the pain becomes too uncomfortable to bear. And doing this over and over again, during a day, a week, a month, a year, will take its toll. The constant reminder to honour this principle, which is not so readily available with many kinds of work, helps the practitioner to avoid the causes of fatigue.

As well as physical posture, there is mental posture too. A Zero Balancing practitioner is taught to hold the client in the highest personal regard. At first sight this might seem to be just a vaguely pleasant, or possibly naively sentimental, exhortation. But it is both easy to do and immensely practical. It is easy because any attitude is a choice: it really is possible to decide to regard another person as a threat or a boon. There is an old saying that your worst enemy is your greatest teacher; even beginning to admit that such a person might be teaching you something brings about a shift in your attitude to him or her. So the practitioner can actively choose to accord her client this level of respect and regard. And it helps a lot that she doesn't have to start the session with the kind of medical diagnosis which – however subtly put – is based on finding out what is wrong with the person. There is nothing wrong with a client of Zero Balancing. He may have pain, or be frustrated in his life's work, or may even have just walked out on his partner. All of this helps create a suitable frame for the session, but there is no need to judge it or regard it as a pathology. The work is the same anyway; it is to find the places of held energy and put a clearer, stronger force field through them. Of course, the practitioner may well believe that if she does so the pain will ease, or even that the impetus or motivation for walking out may weaken. But that belief is not a moral imperative; it is simply based on experience that when people's energy and structure are well-balanced they tend to live their lives in such a way as to bring joy to themselves and those around them.

Finally in this chapter I want to point to the similarities between the practice of Zero Balancing and the practice of meditation. In order to feel the movements of energy in a client's body, the practitioner has to be still herself; if she is moving she will not be able to tell whether the movement she is feeling is hers or the client's. Nor can a fulcrum be held still if she is jittery or restless. There is a strong parallel between this and the stillness of sitting meditation. In both Zero Balancing and meditation, the mind is quiet but attention is very present and focused.

> The practice of meditation is not an exercise in analysis or reasoning... In Vietnam when we cook a pot of dried corn, we concentrate the fire under the pot and several hours later the kernels come loose and split open. When the sun's rays beat down on the snow, the snow slowly melts. When a hen sits on her eggs, the chicks inside gradually take form until they are ready to peck their way out. These are images which illustrate the practice of meditation... (Thich Nhat Hanh, *The Sun My Heart*, p. 29)

Although a Zero Balancing session is rather quicker, these three images capture its spirit nicely. In all of them, it is the focused heat that brings about a transformation; in Zero Balancing, it is the focused attention of the practitioner, as conveyed and expressed in fulcrums, which enables change. The combination of stillness and attention allows a person to live in the present moment; to be fully aware of living and to have a vivid experience of what is happening. Most people assume they are doing that all the time; it is only when, somehow, they actually manage to do it, that they realize what they have been missing.

Working at interface, keeping a donkey connection with the client, and being fully aware of the signs of energetic change require the practitioner to live in the present moment. If her mind is elsewhere, she will be unable to do any of these things, and soon enough, even in that unaware state, she will feel that nothing is happening. In bringing herself back, the rewards are enormous. The client starts to respond again, she feels better, and the atmosphere in the room takes on a quality of charged quietness which is a joy to experience.

Although I have discussed a number of reasons why a practitioner benefits from doing the work, I think it is this last reason which explains why Fritz Smith looked better at the end of ten sessions than he did at the start. He had been in a state of quiet, focused attention, similar to a meditative state, for practically the whole of the day, and had that calm, clear, refreshed presence of a monk. I had always assumed that monks had this quality of being because they were separated from the stresses of jobs and mortgages and children and commuting. But I think that it is more likely that it comes from long periods of meditation – whatever name it is called by different faiths. The Zero Balancing practitioner is in the fortunate position of being able to make her work into a meditation, and her meditation into her work; of making balancing others a way of balancing herself.

developments

· ·

I'm not mystical in spite of being a surgeon; I'm mystical because I'm a surgeon. As a surgeon I watch miracles daily. When I cut the body open I rely on it to heal... The body knows much more than I do. (Bernie S. Siegel MD, *Peace, Love and Healing*, p. 44)

When students of Zero Balancing watch a very experienced and highly skilled practitioner at work, they are often amazed at how little she appears to do. They expect to see all kinds of fancy work – things that were not even referred to in their first workshop, but which they imagine would be taught at advanced level workshops. They are eager to notice unusual fulcrums and departures from the protocol, and anticipate a long session – extra time being needed to incorporate all the sophisticated additions. What they see is quite the opposite. Rarely does the practitioner do anything which isn't taught in the first few days of that first workshop, and the work is over in half the time novice practitioners take to do a session. And what seems extraordinary is that when the client gets up off the couch he looks genuinely revitalized. His eyes are clear and have more sparkle in them. His voice is fuller and firmer, and he walks with more strength and grace. The novice practitioners know that their clients don't usually look as good as this, but they can't spot the magic ingredient; what was it the expert did that made the difference? They can't spot it because they are looking for the wrong thing. It isn't extra work, it is an extra quality of the work.

They are surprised I think, because their experience of education is to keep on learning more; more facts, more concepts, more techniques. But with something that is an art and a skill, expertise is not so much about learning more, but about learning to use the basics better. A master joiner uses the same techniques of woodworking as a skilled apprentice, but the furniture he produces will look right, in some indefinable way, feel better to use, and last longer. Simple Yoga postures, to take another example, can be learned quite quickly, but it takes a lifetime of practice to do them effortlessly and to explore their full potential. Zero Balancing is an art and a skill, and the master does what the novice does, only with a different quality of work, and the results are more profound and longer lasting.

In keeping with the spirit of this, I want to return to a few of the key ideas of Zero Balancing; looking at the way this quality is added, and pointing towards some of the developments of the future – both in the work itself and in the part it may play in the wider world of health care.

. . . .

the fulcrum revisited

I recently gave a session to a middle-aged woman suffering from recurrent neck pain following a whiplash injury some years ago. She is otherwise fit and well; she eats good food and takes plenty of exercise. When I started to work I found that her whole body, including her neck, was strong and flexible; I couldn't find the source of her problems under my hands. Even when I put in a half moon from her head, affecting the whole of her neck, nothing much seemed to happen. Although the fulcrum was technically adequate, somehow I wasn't in touch with the pain nor with whatever it was that was causing it. Then, suddenly, I felt that underneath the flexibility was a tightness – even a rather desperate holding on. I held the fulcrum for a few moments and felt the tightness start to yield. In the space created by that yielding I put in another, tiny, half moon on top of the first – Figure 15 represents this. With that little extra half moon, the fulcrum was right there; doing its work of rebalancing not at the surface level where all was fine, but at the deeper level where it was not.

This fulcrum was near the end of the session. When she came back the next time – her neck feeling a lot better – I was alerted, and found the same pattern in other places too; places where, misled by the surface flexibility, I'd missed it before. At this point it was clear to me that if I worked consistently on the tension underneath the flexibility, the session would have a far more powerful and widespread effect than she might have envisaged. What I was noticing was some aspect of her life, not just some aspect of her body. So I asked her if she wanted to work on this pattern, and she did. From then on, although the fulcrums might have looked the same to an observer, they had a different quality and were operating at a different level than in the first session. At this level, distinctions between body, mind and spirit cannot be maintained. They are consistent aspects of one person, different viewpoints of the same whole; and working on any one aspect will affect all the others. Of course, this isn't my idea, it is as old as human history, and has been said by countless people in countless ways. One poetic version of it is, 'When the tide comes in, all the boats float.'

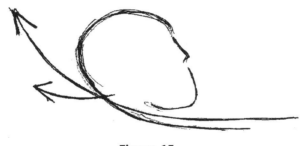

Figure 15

Fulcrums at this level can be seen as having two stages. First, the area where it is applied is taken out of the form it has been in, and then secondly, the fulcrum holds it in a new form for a few moments to allow it to settle and take on that new form. In general terms, this is how things are changed. A horseshoe is made from a straight piece of metal; it is first heated, which releases the forces holding it into that form, and then reshaped to fit the hoof. Relationships, too, have a form. Change takes place when some crisis takes it out of its original form for a period of time; something has to shake the form loose first. Then it will settle into a new form – and those who deliberately create a new form, and hold it, get the new relationship they choose. So, to return to the example of the woman with neck pain, if she is willing to work on the stiffness underneath the flexibility, the fulcrums will create an opportunity for change in her mind and spirit as well as her body.

This may sound alarming. Is it safe? How does the practitioner know what she is doing at these levels? There are a number of reasons for believing it is absolutely safe. Most obviously, the client may have asked for this kind of change at these levels – either before the session starts, as his reason for coming, or when asked during the session. Also, working at interface and with a donkey connection means that the practitioner is not imposing anything of her own on the client; and if her touch feels good or hurts good – as it always should – then the body is welcoming the experience and it can safely be assumed that the mind and spirit are content too.

More specifically, it is an absolutely unmistakable feeling, in the practitioner's hands, when a client is not willing for an area of his body to be taken out of its existing form. As the fulcrum is placed, she can feel quite clearly that there is a resistance – sometimes conscious, more often unconscious – to moving out of form. And she always respects this. There is no judgement of it at all. It is simply not a part of Zero Balancing that the practitioner knows best how the client should be; she puts in the fulcrums which provide an opportunity for change, but if nothing happens she respects that and doesn't try to force one. When, while I was holding the half moon, the space in my client's neck opened up, that was her choice, again consciously or unconsciously, to let go of some of the form she had been holding. I wasn't expecting it; still less demanding it. I was simply paying careful attention, otherwise I would never have felt that opening.

The same holds true for the new form which is established. The practitioner doesn't know how the body will re-organize around the fulcrum and resettle afterwards, and certainly doesn't plan it. Having sensed, through her fingertips, a place which has potential for change, her fulcrum there can be seen as an unspoken question addressed to the client, 'Is this a place where you would like to take the opportunity to re-organize?' Sometimes, the answer is 'No'; and nothing happens. Sometimes it feels more like 'No, thanks'; that is, there is a softening and easing around the fulcrum, but no real change. But if the answer is an unequivocal 'Yes', she will feel the shift under her fingers and hold the fulcrum until she realizes, by a sign from the client, that it has finished its work. It is an example of 'the dance' I referred to in the last chapter. At this part of the dance, the client is leading. And the direction in which he is leading is not set by his will or his intention; it is an innate response. That is really why it is safe. There is an increasingly voluminous literature, by doctors such as Andrew Weil and psychotherapists such as Carl Rogers, which all affirm the innate disposition of the body and mind to heal itself.

The way in which Zero Balancing has developed leads me to the same conclusion too. Initially, Fritz Smith's medical practice was in a rural area, and he used Zero Balancing to help relieve musculo-skeletal pain, and back pain in particular. After some years of this kind of work he noticed that it was having wider and deeper effects on his patients. People who came for treatment feeling dull, listless and ill at ease with themselves and their lives became more positive in their outlook, and started to relate better to their families and colleagues. Those who were going through particularly stressful times seemed to manage the stress better, and indeed to use it as an opportunity to become clearer about what they really wanted from their lives. At first, I imagine these outcomes were seen as benign side effects of the work; but eventually they could no longer be passed off in this way. More and more patients were coming precisely for these side effects and they were getting what they came for, reliably and regularly. It was not that Fritz Smith set out to revitalize his patients' minds and spirits, rather that it was no longer possible to deny that the work was having these effects. In this respect, theory followed clinical results.

So a new cycle of theory and practice was set up. Given that the work could provide these opportunities, how could the practitioner's technique and skills make the most of them? The answer to that question has two aspects. Partly, it is a matter of refining the quality of attention. In the early stages of learning Zero Balancing, the practitioner's attention will be focused on being able to recognize the sensation of held energy under her fingertips; then it will be on the kind of fulcrum which will help to release that held energy. With experience, she starts to be able to feel the client's energy body as a whole, and to notice its state. In one of my clients, the energy body has a buzzing, over-stimulated, high revving quality, rather like a car being driven fast in second gear. The feeling I have is that if he could only change gear, he could do more with much less effort. Another client's energy body, by contrast, feels exhausted, flat and empty – to use the car image again, it is as if he is coasting along in neutral because he knows he has very little fuel left in his tank. Figure 16 (a) and (b) show visually the energy bodies of the two clients I have described.

As you would expect, the first client becomes very anxious about what, even to him, are small things, and finds it hard to relax and to go to sleep. The second client would like to care more than he does about the events of his life and to have more power and determination to get what he wants – most of the time he can't quite be bothered to seize opportunities or to do what he knows would help his health and happiness. Interestingly, the first client's voice is quick, sharp and vibrant, whereas the second client's is dull and monotonous – irrespective of the content of what they are saying. The tone, timbre and quality of the sound they each make is completely different; it has a different vibration. This concept of vibration provides a language for representing and talking about the energy body.

Carolyn Myss, whose accuracy in diagnosing disease by intuition has been confirmed, after extensive evaluation, by Norman Shealy MD, writes, 'each illness and each body organ, I learned, has its own "frequency" or vibrational pattern...' She adds, 'I believe that all tissues hold the vibrational patterns of our attitudes, our belief systems...' (Caroline Myss, *Anatomy of the Spirit*, pp. 22, 26).

Similarly, Valerie Hunt, a renowned neurophysiologist, writes, 'If the healing response is automatic...then what goes wrong when healing does not occur? ...the problem is in the flow of electro-magnetic energy, its strength and range of vibrations, as well as its coherency' (Valerie V. Hunt, *Infinite Mind*, p. 257).

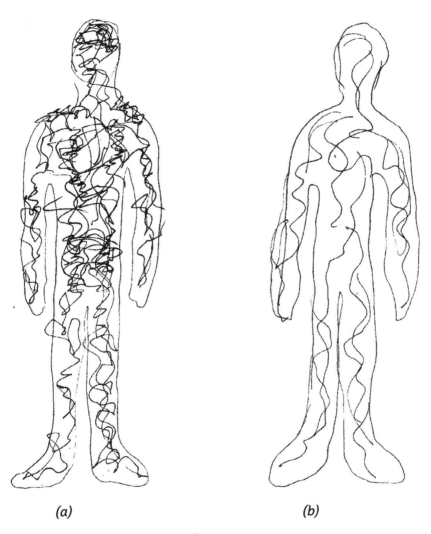

(a) *(b)*

Figure 16

It is easiest to apply these kinds of insights to Zero Balancing if I go right back to basics. The essential method is to put a clearer, stronger force field through a bone or joint; one which overrides the existing force field which is holding energy and structure in its current unbalanced state. A fulcrum is simply the technique for doing that. So it is a small step to suggest that a clearer, stronger force field, not just through a bone or joint but through the existing whole energy body, changing its vibration, will be of benefit to both the people I have referred to above. The fascinating question is, 'How can a fulcrum be put through an entire energy body?'

To some extent, over a whole session, a series of fulcrums in different parts of the body will have an effect on the general vibration of the client's energy body. But, given a practised level of attention, the practitioner can work more specifically and deliberately than that. She can put in a fulcrum to affect the vibration itself. One way of doing this is by building a fulcrum on a fulcrum, in the way I described earlier with the half moon on my client's neck. With the first fulcrum, energy and structure are held in a state of balance at one location. As soon as they are in balance there, the practitioner's fingers are no longer receiving messages about the imbalance at one particular place and she can feel the vibration of the whole energy body under her fingertips. Holding a state of balance in one place allows her to sense the nature of the whole; in fact, she is literally in touch with it. So if she then adds another fulcrum it will have a direct effect on that general vibration. It may sound a little abstract, but what is happening is that she is putting a fulcrum into the vibration – she is holding it under her fingers and providing a still point around which it can re-organize.

I want to emphasize that, as usual, the practitioner has no particular intention when she places fulcrums of this kind; they simply provide an opportunity for reorganization. She may expect, to take the example of Figure 16 (a), that the effect of the fulcrum will be to calm and settle the agitation, but she is not disappointed or critical if it doesn't. Her attention will have led her to notice what is there and to put in a fulcrum, but that doesn't mean that she wants it to be different. She wants it to be as the client chooses it to be, and the fulcrum provides access to choices which he may not have had before.

All this is a long way from the initial picture of Zero Balancing painted in the first chapter. The journey is the same as that taken by Fritz Smith, and the practitioners who have learned from him. Briefly, it starts as a way of working easily and effectively on musculo-skeletal problems; using the theory that balancing energy and structure opens up a route to healing. Then it gradually becomes clear that particular areas of the body hold certain kinds of memories and emotions, and the work starts to have wider effects. With more experience, improvements in the mental and spiritual well-being of clients become common, and the basic techniques are refined to reach these more directly. The potential of the fulcrum has expanded, and continues to expand. At each stage there is a delay between what Fritz Smith finds he can do in practice and his ability to describe and explain it. This is not surprising. What is surprising is that he has been able to communicate so clearly what he actually does – finding concepts such as interface, donkey and fulcrums to describe the way he responds, through touch, to what he knows will serve his clients. In addition, he has also been able to explain, in the provisional way appropriate to all theories, why it works. He is currently working in ways and at levels which neither he nor I can yet fully describe or explain. The developments continue.

the context

As outlined in Chapter 1, it has been simplest to write about Zero Balancing in isolation, as if it were a self-contained set of ideas and a unique form of therapy. In fact, it is a product of its time, both arising from and contributing to an enormous cultural change in medicine and health care. This change involves, at least, new perceptions of the body, of the role of doctors, of medicine and of the nature of healing. I want to outline this cultural change in order to put Zero Balancing in its proper context, and to give some indication of the ways in which it, and medicine in general, may develop in the future.

First comes an increasing sensitivity to the relationship of mind and body, and to the part played by the mind in healing the body. Andrew Weil, a doctor, tells this story of his wife's pregnancy.

Three weeks before Sabine's due date I asked a friend and colleague, Dr Steve Gurgevich, who practises hypnotherapy, to do a session with her, again in the interests of a timely, quick, uncomplicated birth. The baby was in a posterior presentation at this time, which worried us. Sabine's last baby had been posterior, causing long, painful labor. Steve did an hour long session with her at the end of an afternoon, encouraging Sabine to talk with the baby, asking her to turn round before the beginning of labor and help make the labor quick. When he brought Sabine out of her reverie, she looked supremely relaxed. After Steve left, Sabine and I went into the kitchen to start dinner. Suddenly she clutched her belly and bent over.

'What is it?' I asked.

'I think the baby's turning,' she said, amazed.

It happened that our midwife was coming to dinner that night. She examined Sabine and reported that the baby was now in an anterior presentation, having turned within 20 minutes of being asked to do so. The baby came right on her due date, October 4. Labor lasted a mere two hours and six minutes, which was, if anything, a little too brief in that we barely had time to prepare... I see a clear role of the mind in healing, visible in correlations of healing responses with mental and emotional changes. (Andrew Weil MD, *Spontaneous Healing*, pp. 99–100)

Bernie Siegel, a surgeon, writes, 'Years of experience have taught me that cancer and indeed nearly all diseases are psychosomatic. This may sound strange to people accustomed to thinking that psychosomatic ailments are not truly "real", but believe me they are' (Bernie S. Siegel MD, *Love, Medicine and Miracles*, p. 111).

Deepak Chopra MD makes the same point in a more philosophical vein, 'Because Western medicine assumes that a person is a physical machine who happens to think, we find ourselves out on a limb, a naked spur of history. The great traditions of wisdom, embracing medicine, philosophy, psychology and religion, have all believed exactly the opposite: we are thoughts that have learned to create a physical machine' (Richard Carlson and Benjamin Shield (eds.), *Healers on Healing*, p. 181).

A different angle on this is provided by research into the performance of top class athletes. They have a term for a state of being when it seems that they can do no wrong; they know they can hit the ball wherever they want whenever they want, however fast it comes to them; they know they are going to jump over the pole, even though it is higher than they have ever jumped before. They call it being in 'the zone'. It is a curious combination of deep relaxation with acute concentration and awareness. Researchers have monitored patterns of brain activity while athletes are in the zone and discovered that the normal patterns are replaced by what they call alpha waves; and that exactly the same pattern of alpha waves is observed in people in a deep state of meditation.

All of this applies to Zero Balancing too. During a session, the client will often fall into that state of deep relaxation and awareness which characterizes the zone; and it sounds like the state in which Sabine Weil was able to talk to her baby – her husband reported that she looked 'supremely relaxed' after her session. So it is not fanciful to suppose that a Zero Balancing session can help the client to regain mental clarity or emotional stability, and manage better the problems and issues he is finding difficult in his life.

Receiving touch at interface, to take another example, conveys a strong message to the mind – 'touch can be safe' – and it is obvious that this may do much to change the mental perceptions of those who have suffered from abusive or insensitive touch in the past. It may allow them to accept, and eventually welcome, touch in intimate relationships and will play a part in healing any physical or emotional wounds inflicted by the abuse. More generally, a prolonged donkey connection will affect the mind. With a client who feels unsupported in his life, it can convey a message to the mind that he can receive support at the same time as giving him a body-felt sensation of support which validates and reinforces the message. He may have learned to doubt or mistrust words such as 'I support you', creating mental confusion and uncertainty when support is offered in ordinary life. But, in a session, his donkey will know whether or not the feeling of being supported is true. And then, most obviously, there are the words a practitioner uses. The frame, at the start of the session, gives a clear and positive invitation to the mind to set about resolving whatever it was that brought the client for help. Talking during a session can be even more powerful. Very experienced practitioners (novices are warned, and should recognize, this is such a powerful intervention that it requires great skill) will sometimes make suggestions to the client which amplify the message being conveyed by their hands. One phrase that Fritz Smith uses often is, 'Let drop away anything which no longer serves you', while at the same time holding the whole rib cage with one strong and reassuring fulcrum. And the effect is that the client's mind and body can co-operate in releasing both mental patterns and body-held memories simultaneously. Working explicitly with the mind is one aspect of Zero Balancing which Fritz Smith is developing intensively.

This integration of mind and body is but one part of a larger re-perception. Valerie Hunt spent the latter part of her distinguished career doing scientific research on energy fields in the body. She writes, 'Electromedical researchers believe that each disease or functional disturbance has its own energy field which must be reversed before healing can take place. Probably illness is a disturbance first in the energy field and healing is the restoration of that field to health. Soon we should be able to show unequivocally that field disturbance precedes all tissue change' (Valerie V. Hunt, *Infinite Mind*, p. 244).

Her work follows the lead, given long before, by Albert Einstein. He wrote, 'We may regard matter as being constituted by the regions of space in which the field is extremely intense... There is no place in this new kind of physics both for the field and matter, for the field is the only reality' (Albert Einstein in Arnold Mindell, *Dreambody*, p. 15).

You may have wondered, earlier in the book, 'Does it really make sense to talk about held energy in the bone?' But if bone is just a relatively dense or intense field, then in some places it is likely to be more dense than others. Sounds the same, to me, as held energy. And if held energy in bone is a field, rather than – as we normally imagine – something immutably solid, then it begins to look much more plausible that it can change quite quickly. And the blindingly obvious way to change an existing field is by putting a clearer, stronger one through it.

It is not just one bone that is a field, so is the whole body. Earlier in this chapter, I described the way a skilled practitioner can put a fulcrum into the vibration of the body as a whole – and commented that the idea might sound a little abstract. In the light of this physics, it is really no more abstract than putting a fulcrum into a bone. To be sure, it is easier to feel the dense field of a bone than the more diffuse field in which the body exists; but it doesn't take very long to learn. In fact, I suspect that we are a lot better at it than we give ourselves credit for. How often have you felt a person was standing, somehow, a bit too close to you for comfort? Surely an indication that you actually felt that person entering your field. And how often have you known, but not known how you knew, that someone was lying, troubled, ill, or indeed, supremely well and clear? These may well have been qualities of their field which you were sensing quickly and accurately.

It is informative to describe the development of Zero Balancing in terms of fields. It started by working on the localized fields of particular places in bones and joints, where that field was felt as unclear or incoherent. (Notice that in talking of fields, it no longer makes much sense to distinguish energy and structure – they are simply convenient ways of describing the field from different points of view.) A change in the field produced a change in the functioning of the body. Then it was realized that these local interventions were having an effect on the larger field; one which certainly included the mind as well as the body, so the work developed in ways which addressed the larger field itself. At this level of work, the purpose and outcome of a session may be to restore a client's self-esteem or to stimulate his creativity or provide him with an experience of himself unaffected by the turmoil of major upheavals in his life. This kind of work may lead to the sort of profound and lasting changes normally thought possible only through prolonged and intensive psychotherapy or spiritual practices, with changes in chronic physical ailments possible as a consequence, too. Fritz Smith is, intuitively, working with fields in ways beyond anything I can grasp, let alone report here.

Another aspect of this is a re-perception of healing. The focus of Western medicine is on the elimination of pathology. A person has symptoms which are painful, unpleasant, even life-threatening, and the doctor's job is to remove or alleviate them. Countless patients have good reason to be grateful to this form of medicine and those who practise it, and I have no doubt that it will long continue to provide the major source of health care in modern society. However, in the past 20 years or so, along with extraordinary developments in the scope of this form of medicine, there has arisen a different perspective. To take one example, not long ago the removal or alleviation of a symptom would have been taken as synonymous with healing; now, in the words of a famous osteopath, who writes from this new perspective, 'true healing goes deeper than symptoms...healing may sometimes mean spending the rest of your life in a wheelchair...the successful therapeutic process does not necessarily produce comfort, ease, muscular strength, prolonged life, or any of the other things that our Western medical tradition has come to hold as evidence of healing' (Richard Carlson and Benjamin Shield (eds.), *Healers on Healing*, pp. 71–72).

It is hard to imagine such sentiments being expressed 20 years ago by someone with a conventional medical training, and I am sure that some readers will still find them puzzling, even disturbing. Most dramatic of all is the title of a book by a well-known teacher and author Stephen Levine, *Healing into Life and Death*.

This is a large topic and I want to mention just two aspects of it. The first is that, according to this perspective, healing is not something which any person can do to another – let alone any doctor or therapist. Healing is a natural process of what I will now call the bodymind, which can only be helped or hindered, but not done, by outside intervention. Bernie Siegel writes, 'I have to try to remember that I am merely a facilitator of healing, not the healer himself...' (Bernie S. Siegel MD, *Peace, Love and Healing*, p. 145).

This is, of course, the same view that lies behind the emphasis in Zero Balancing on putting in a fulcrum without intention and allowing the body to re-organize around it. The practitioner creates opportunities and possibilities which may not have been open to the client before, and leaves it to him to choose – consciously or unconsciously – whether or not to take them. As is clear from both his books, Bernie Siegel sees surgery in just this light; the removal of a cancerous tumour does not heal the patient, but it may provide an opportunity for him to heal. In the terms I have just used, the surgery can be seen as a fulcrum into the field.

The other aspect of this issue hinges on expectations. In an experiment, people were shown a number of playing cards, one after the other and asked to simply say what card they saw. In among the cards were some anomalies – for example a seven with a spade shape, but the shape was coloured red and not black; or a five with a heart shape coloured black rather than red. Hardly any of the subjects reported the card accurately. Most of them, expecting the spade shape to be black or the heart shape to be red, reported that the cards were simply the seven of spades and the five of hearts.

Similarly seeing a person who is suffering from acute pain, enormous disability or a life-threatening illness, most people report that the person is suffering badly. However, there are countless stories of anomalies – the books I have quoted from are full of them; stories of patients in just these circumstances who are happy and who communicate joy to all those who have the privilege of being with them. It is only recently that doctors, and indeed friends and relations, have managed to alter their expectations sufficiently to see the happiness and joy in the midst of pain. And to be able to say of such people that they have healed notwithstanding their symptoms. Equally, there are plenty of people who, according to all the medical tests, have no identifiable disease or illness, but who feel wretched and despair of life, who are not healed. Stephen Levine, who has spent many years with people who are dying, writes about those who recovered from apparently fatal illnesses, 'the healing of the body for many was a by-product of a new balance of mind and heart. It wasn't that these people felt better than ever because they had healed, but rather that they had healed because they had come upon a place of a bit more ease and peace within' (Stephen Levine, *Healing into Life and Death*, p. 4).

This is the experience, too, of clients and practitioners of Zero Balancing. On the one hand, when symptoms do disappear and pain is relieved, it seems to be a consequence of the inner calm that clients feel both during and after a session. One piece of evidence for this is that, quite often, especially in the case of chronic pain, there may be no change for a day or two, and then it gradually starts to fade away. So it cannot be that the calm is the result of an easing of pain. Once again, it seems to be the change in the field that does the work, and the patterns of the body respond a little more slowly than the patterns of the mind.

It is also the case that for some clients there is no noticeable improvement in specific symptoms. For some of them, this is a disappointment, and indeed the work has not helped. However, a good many report the same kind of healing that is referred to in the books I have quoted. A renewed zest for life makes it possible to enjoy each day in spite of the persistence of symptoms which were, when the world seemed a grey place, intolerable. In conventional medical thinking, the fact that the symptoms persisted would be proof that the therapy isn't working; but from this new perspective, that is too narrow a definition of 'working'. People can bear all sorts of discomfort with equanimity if their spirits are high.

It may be a minor example, but I can't help thinking of a client I worked with recently. A middle-aged woman, she was desperately depressed by her size and weight, which were well above average. For many years she had tried one slimming regime after another, really tried, but the few pounds she had lost with each of them had soon gone back on. She saw herself as an unlovely and unlovable lump, lumbering around like a hippopotamus. After a few sessions she hadn't lost any weight, but she moved with grace and dignity, carrying her weight easily. She said she felt like a dancer, and she looked radiant. Seeing herself in that way she began to expect others to see herself in that way too, and they did. Nothing was cured, but a lot was healed.

. . . .

keeping it simple

For all the explorations of this chapter, the basic ideas of Zero Balancing are very simple. Although it may take a lifetime to master them, everyone who is involved in health care can learn from them. Touching at interface, and making a donkey connection with the person who is being touched, can provide a safe and comforting connection with another human being, which so many who are suffering want so badly. The stillness of a held fulcrum, and the pause after it, can give a client a few moments away from the personality which has been moulded and distorted by the pressures of his upbringing and his life, a few moments when he can feel truly himself. A practitioner, working with real attention, without intending or expecting a particular change in the client, conveys a deep message that he is accepted, recognized and appreciated as he is. These are fundamental to healing; indeed they are fundamental to any genuine contact with another person. They can be given to any patient or client, whether or not they ever have a Zero Balancing session. And the person who provides them will receive the gifts of them too, in abundance.

bibliography

Ackroyd, Peter, *Blake*, London: Minerva, 1996.

Becker, Robert O. and Selden, Gary, *The Body Electric*, New York: Quill Books, 1985.

Carlson, Richard and Shield, Benjamin (eds.), *Healers on Healing*, Los Angeles: Jeremy P. Tarcher Inc., 1989.

Dass, Ram and Gorman, Paul, *How Can I Help?*, London: Rider, 1986.

Hanh, Thich Nhat, *The Sun My Heart*, Berkley, California: Parallax Press, 1988.

Heller, Joseph, *Catch 22*, London: Corgi, 1964.

Hunt, Valerie V., *Infinite Mind*, Malibu: Malibu Publishing, 1989.

James, William, *Varieties of Religious Experience*, London and Glasgow: Fontana, 1974.

Levine, Stephen, *Healing into Life and Death*, Bath: Gateway Books, 1989.

Mindell, Arnold, *Dreambody*, London: Arkana, 1990.

Mitchell, Stephen (tr.), *Tao Te Ching*, New York: Harper Perennial, 1988.

Myss, Caroline, *Anatomy of the Spirit*, New York: Bantam, 1997.

Palmer, William A. (ed.), *J.S. Bach*, California: Alfred Publishing, 1983.

Pert, Candace, *Molecules of Emotion*, New York: Scribner, 1997.

Rodegast, Pat and Stanton, Judith (eds.), *Emmanuel's Book: A Manual for Living Comfortably in the Cosmos*, New York: Bantam, 1987.

Sacks, Dr Oliver, *A Leg to Stand On*, London: Picador, 1991.

Siegel MD, Bernie S., *Love, Medicine and Miracles*, London: Arrow, 1988.

Siegel MD, Bernie S., *Peace, Love and Healing*, London: Arrow, 1990.

Smith MD, Fritz Frederick, *Inner Bridges*, Atlanta: Humanics, 1986.

Suzuki, Shunryu, *Zen Mind, Beginner's Mind*, New York: Weatherhill, 1970.

Weil MD, Andrew, *Spontaneous Healing*, New York: Fawcett Columbine, 1996.

Wilber, Ken, *Sex, Ecology, Spirituality*, Boston: Shambala, 1995.

useful addresses

For details about certified Zero Balancing practitioners, or to find out about the workshops and courses that are being offered, you can contact the Zero Balancing Association:

uk

Zero Balancing Association UK
Membership Office
21 Ivy Road
Stirchley, Birmingham B30 2NU
Telephone: 0845 603 6805
Email: info@zerobalancinguk.org
Website: www.zerobalancinguk.org

italy

Zero Balancing Italy
Email: info@zerobalancing.it
Website: www.zerobalancing.it

spain

Zero Balancing Spain
Telephone: 93 848 20 73
Email: info@zerobalancing.es
Website: www.zerobalancing.es

switzerland

Zero Balancing Association (Switzerland)
c/o practice for body therapy
Waidstrasse 17
CH-8037 Zurich
Telephone: 41 0 272 78 81
Email: info@zerobalancing.ch
Website: www.zerobalancing.ch

us

Zero Balancing Health Association
8640 Guilford Road, Suite 241
Columbia, MD 21046 USA
Telephone: 410 381 8956
Website: www.zerobalancing.com

mexico

Zero Balancing Mexico
Netzahualcoyotl No.1
Tepoztlan, Morelos
Mexico CP62520
Telephone: 01 739 395 1377
Email: Balanceceromexico@prodigy.net.mx
Website: www.balanceceromexico.com

new zealand/australia

The Zero Balancing Association New Zealand/Australia
PO Box 682
Onera, Waiheke Island 1081, New Zealand
Telephone: 64 9 372 3115
Email: zbanza@xtra.co.nz
Website: www.zerobalancing.co.nz

index

Made in the USA
Middletown, DE
07 December 2019